Praise fo

"Len Lantz shares solid, quality help in a befriending, relational, and conversational manner. His humorous illustrations and real stories make this serious subject engaging and approachable. Get it, read it, use it. It will make a genuine difference for you and for God's kingdom!"

—**DOUGLAS DIEHL**, retired United Methodist pastor

"Len has an important message to those who for too long have labeled depression as taboo or due to a lack of faith or persevering. . . . I will be sure to recommend *unJoy* to those struggling with depression and invite them onto the path of recovery that Len lays out. Well done, Dr. Lantz!"

—**ERIC KRONER**, TEAM missionary in Chad, Africa

"*UnJoy* is a book that brings hope. As a pastor of more than thirty-eight years, I've seen too many Christ followers struggle with the stigma of guilt and shame as they live under the dark cloud of depression. I wish I could have given them this book. . . . If you struggle with depression or love and care for someone who does, this book is for you."

—**CHRIS DOLSON**, pastor emeritus, Blackhawk Church

"Being a Christian doesn't mean being immune from depression, but for many, it's easier to see a doctor to fix a broken bone or even treat cancer than to address a mental health concern. Dr. Lantz shows how people of faith can find relief from depression through a variety of therapies. If you think you might be depressed—or know someone who is—read this book. It could change your life."

—**MATT RANDLES**, author of *Deep Focus*

"This important book will empower more Christians to move past the stigma associated with mental illness and seek help from a caring and competent professional who can be a guardian of hope sent by God. I found the reflections at the end of each chapter particularly helpful."

—**CHRISTOPHER FULLER, PhD**, theologian

"Dr. Lantz offers the perfect combination of compassion, humor, and expertise to deliver a message of hope and real solutions for depression. This is *lifesaving* information that is desperately needed in today's world."

—**ERIN AMATO, MD**, psychiatrist

"This book is effortless to read and incredibly easy to understand. Len has balanced his medical expertise and Christian faith well, making them neither obtuse nor heavy-handed in considering the subject of depression. . . . How incredibly helpful this book will be for Christians in overcoming depression!"

—**KERMIT CULVER**, retired pastor

"Len Lantz's *unJoy* is a joy for all who read it, whether they are depressed or not. . . . Len got it right: 'This is not a self-help book. It is a get-help book.' Effective treatment shortens distress and dysfunction caused by depression and reduces the risk of recurrence. As a Christian physician with decades of experience treating depression, I see tremendous value in this book."

—**JOHN GREIST, MD**, coauthor of *Depression and Its Treatment*

"*UnJoy* is the real deal, with helpful, understandable, to-the-point information for those struggling with depression. I can't wait to share this book with my Christian family member who is struggling with depression."

—**SCOTT POLAND**, psychologist and suicide prevention expert

"Len Lantz directly addresses so many of the fears and stereotypes that depressed people, Christian and non-Christian alike, experience on a day-to-day basis. Not only does he provide the most recent strategies and interventions, but he does a masterful job of explaining in terms that all of us can understand. This book should be provided to every person experiencing depression as a way of countering the stigma that stops so many from getting help."

—**KARL ROSSTON, LCSW**, psychotherapist

"In *unJoy*, Len Lantz contributes beautifully to an effectual dialogue that neither replaces nor contradicts faith or Scripture. He brings a vibrant, practical humanity to our common struggles with depression. Please read and share *unJoy* with your friends and colleagues!"

—**KEVIN HADDUCK**, author of *A Farewell to Lent*

"*UnJoy* is a fantastic read! Stop waiting with your silent pain and suffering and get this book for yourself or a loved one. Len Lantz has created an amazing resource that is easy and enjoyable to read and also well supported by research. I can see using *unJoy* to help my Christian patients in the treatment of their depression."

—**JENNIFER PREBLE, LCSW**, suicide prevention advocate

"Len Lantz's experience, efforts, and ministry in the world of mental health are well established. The ideas he presents in *unJoy* are straightforward, understandable, and actionable. . . . Len helps remove the stigma around mental health and makes it easier for people to get the help they need. I'll be handing this book to people in my church and community."

—**KEITH JOHNSON**, senior pastor, Life Covenant Church

"Dr. Lantz embraces his faith and psychiatric expertise to offer an easy-to-read book that guides you and your loved ones to find help to conquer 'unJoy.' . . . Dr. Lantz's wise guidance paves the way for compassionate and common-sense treatments that will reduce suffering, help heal depression, and save lives. Read *unJoy*! Give this book to those who need hope and relief from depression."

—**KEITH FOSTER, MD**, child and adolescent psychiatrist

"I am so thankful for this book that joins the wisdom of psychiatry and the heart of the gospel hand in hand to help people comprehensively flourish. What I am looking forward to the most as a pastor is getting this book in the hands of those I care for who have 'an inability to experience pleasure from activities that usually are enjoyable; a loss of joy.' Thank you, Dr. Lantz!"

—**SETH DOMBACH**, lead pastor, Headwaters Covenant Church

"*UnJoy* is a gift to all Christians struggling with their mental health. I have had the honor of being Len's colleague and friend for over a decade. Len Lantz is passionate about helping people with depression. . . . *UnJoy* is the first book that I have encountered that seamlessly pulls together Christianity and mental health. I absolutely plan to buy and share this book with my Christian patients."

—**HEATHER ZALUSKI, MD**, child and adolescent psychiatrist

"Len Lantz has hit a home run with his book *unJoy*! Aligning the medical treatment of depression with Christian principles, Dr. Lantz writes from the perspective of his own strong Christian faith, combined with his medical/psychiatric expertise, and all through the lens of his compassionate care as a wise and experienced healer."

—**JOHN BATTAGLIA, MD**, author of *Doing Supportive Psychotherapy*

"Dr. Len Lantz is a leader in the field of psychiatry and suicide prevention. His Christian faith and medical expertise join together in *unJoy*, the perfect guide to help Christians in their journey with depression."

—**MATT KUNTZ**, executive director, NAMI Montana

"*UnJoy* reveals a compassionate, evidence-based approach to conquering stigma for Christians with depression. He presents a warm, optimistic plan to help Christians overcome their own biases and fears about depression and to be able to get the treatment that they need and deserve. . . . I will definitely be recommending this book to my Christian patients, and it will have a home on my office bookshelf!"

—**JOAN M. GREEN, MD**, child and adolescent psychiatrist

"'The doctor is in!' *UnJoy* is informative, inspired, and insightful. Dr. Len Lantz tells us how to move from 'unJoy' to the joyfulness that is possible through hope and healing."

—**DONALD T. ROBINSON**, North Park Theological Seminary

"*UnJoy* is a comprehensive and easy-to-understand book about depression for Christians and non-Christians alike. . . . I will definitely recommend this book to my clients and other practitioners!"

—**JOAN FITZGERALD, LCSW**, mental health provider

"*UnJoy* is one of the most informative books I have ever read on depression, its causes, and effective treatments. . . . *UnJoy* is a step toward ending the stigma and isolation that has prevented many Christians from accessing effective help."

—**GARY MIHELISH**, past president, NAMI Montana

unJoy

unJoy

Hope and Help for 7 Million Christians with Depression

LEN LANTZ, MD

RESOURCE *Publications* · Eugene, Oregon

Resource Publications
An Imprint of Wipf and Stock Publishers
199 W. 8th Ave., Suite 3
Eugene, OR 97401

www.wipfandstock.com

PAPERBACK ISBN: 978-1-6667-3546-8
HARDCOVER ISBN: 978-1-6667-9256-0
EBOOK ISBN: 978-1-6667-9257-7

04/25/22

Scriptures taken from the Holy Bible, New International Version®, NIV®. Copyright © 1973, 1978, 1984, 2011 by Biblica, Inc.™ Used by permission of Zondervan. All rights reserved worldwide. www.zondervan.com The "NIV" and "New International Version" are trademarks registered in the United States Patent and Trademark Office by Biblica, Inc.™

This book is designed to provide accurate information to the reader regarding the subject matter. However, neither the publisher nor the author is engaged in rendering professional advice or services to the individual reader. The information presented here is intended to drive discussions between the reader and their healthcare provider and is not intended to diagnose health problems or to replace professional medical care, nor should it be considered a substitute for seeing a physician.

This book is dedicated to my wife Krista
and my daughter Lucy.
You bring me joy.

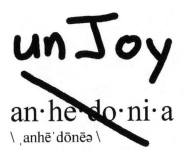

unJoy

an·he·do·ni·a
\ ˌanhēˈdōnēə \

noun **PSYCHIATRY**

1. An inability to experience pleasure from activities that usually are enjoyable.

2. The loss of joy.

Contents

Acknowledgments

YOU PROBABLY KNOW THAT gems don't really shine without a lot of polishing. Well, the same is true for my writing! I'm not sure that I would have had the confidence to write this book or publish any articles without the support of my daughter Lucy and wife Krista. They have both spent a great deal of time polishing my words to make me a better writer and, frankly, polishing *me* to make me a better man, father, and husband. Thank you, Lucy and Krista.

I also want to thank my friends, family, colleagues, and patients who have shared their stories and their lives with me. My life has been enriched by you, and I hope that I have honored your trust and your stories in this book.

I have deep gratitude for the many scientists and researchers who are working to better understand the brain, the causes of depression, treatments for depression, and approaches for preventing suicide. Because of your hard work and dedication, I was able to share many effective strategies for depression in this book. Your work saves lives.

I would also like to provide special thanks to Drs. Barbara Stanley and Greg Brown for permission to use the Safety Planning Intervention form in this book and to Dr. Robert M. A. Hirschfeld for permission to use the Mood Disorder Questionnaire. Thank you for your generosity, passion, and amazing work!

Acknowledgments

I want to thank the many newsletter subscribers of *The Psychiatry Resource* who have read my articles and provided me valuable feedback over the years. I am inspired to hear from you and I love learning from you, too.

Lastly, thank you, Matt Wimer and team at Wipf and Stock Publishers, for giving me and this book a chance. It's not easy to find a home for a book like *unJoy* that spans so many genres: psychiatry, spirituality, counseling, ministry, wellness, and suicide prevention. My prayer is that *unJoy* will be a source of encouragement and a valuable resource for any Christian who is suffering from depression and for those who care for them. Thank you, Matt and team, for helping to make this happen!

Introduction

A Christian Book on Depression with Real Solutions

You make known to me the path of life; you will fill me with joy in your presence, with eternal pleasures at your right hand. (Psalm 16:11)

What's unJoy? (And What's Up with the Bad Drawings?)

I KNOW. I'M MAKING up words and creating scribbles. I was going to say that my artistic ability is that of a preschooler, but, frankly, most preschoolers are better artists than me. All will be explained shortly.

I first want to take just a moment and thank you for opening this book and reading it. Time is a precious commodity, so I've made this book as short and as interesting as possible. I am an expert in treating depression, and I felt called to write something positive and helpful for the many Christians (and their families and friends) who struggle with depression.

You might expect a book on depression to be sad and boring. Well, I didn't want to write a sad and boring book. I want people to have hope, laughter, and freedom from their depression. So I decided to get most of the negative information about depression out of the way in this introduction.

After this introduction, the rest of this book is about solutions, what works to get rid of depression.

The word "unJoy" captures depression in a nutshell. People with depression are often sad or angry when the world around them is just fine or even great! They have a *loss of joy*, which is the most common feature of depression. If you experience unJoy or know someone who does, I hope that you will finish reading this book.

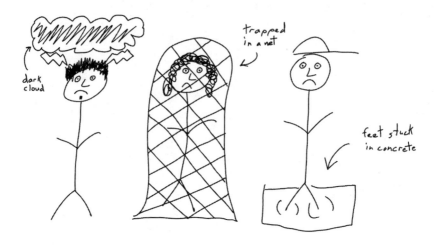

What it can feel like to experience unJoy.

And the bad drawings? I don't intentionally make my drawings terrible—it's just my own natural style (or artistic inability). I happen to like drawings in books, and I have found over time that my family and friends really enjoy my horrible drawings. I hope you do, too! Often, my art is so bad that I have to explain what I drew, so I'll do that when it's needed.

Now, let's look at the problem so that we can move on to the solutions.

What If I Told You That Seven Million Christians across the United States Have Depression Every Year?[1]

Would you believe me? By the way, I'm not talking about all people who identify as Christian. I'm referring to Christians who attend worship services at least once or twice per month.

I find the sheer number of *seven million* Christians with depression to be staggering because I understand how much suffering depression causes people. The number "seven million" also takes my breath away because

---

1. Lantz, "Stigma and 7 Million Christians with Depression."

many of these Christians who are depressed are not reaching out for effective treatment and instead are continuing to suffer.

Please don't be discouraged by that number. There is help and hope for depression, which is what this book is about. And you don't have to be depressed to benefit from this book! This book will help you support others with depression. I wrote this book to convince Christians that:

- Depression and emotional pain are real.
- Strong Christians can still struggle with powerful depression.
- Stigma in the church creates barriers to getting better.
- There are many effective treatments for depression.
- You don't have to suffer from unJoy.

Depression is a serious problem for Christian leaders, congregations, families, and their communities. This problem has been worsened by increasing depression and associated suicide rates each year. Depression is the leading cause of suicide, responsible for up to 70 percent of completed suicides;[2] therefore, addressing depression is one of the most strategic approaches to prevent suicide.

Why Are We as Christians Struggling So Much with Depression?

The problem of depression among Christians is intensified by stigma, which is higher among Christians, especially in certain denominations. Stigma can result in a delay in seeking professional treatment. For example, one of my relatives—I'll call her Sarah—needed acute psychiatric hospitalization because she had struggled alone for years with severe depression, which finally became out of control. When the psychiatric nurse learned that she was a Christian, the nurse exclaimed, "Oh! You must be Baptist!," a statement that startled Sarah with its accuracy.

One out of five people experiences depression in their lifetime. Even though depression is very common, Christians often try to hide it from others due to stigma.

---

2. Takahashi, "Depression and Suicide," 359–60.

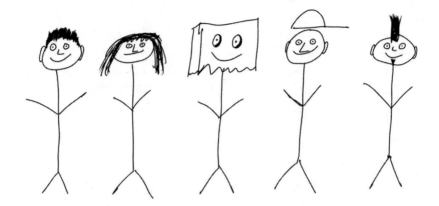

The person in the middle is trying to hide their depression by
wearing a paper bag over their head. They drew a smile on the
bag, which is not a very effective solution for depression.

Stigma results in fear, shame, hiding problems, and not accessing
treatments that alleviate depression. Make no mistake, there is significant
mental health stigma in the Christian church.[3] Research shows that:

- 65 percent of family members related to someone with mental illness
  believe local churches should talk more openly about mental illness to
  reduce stigma.

- 20 percent of individuals with acute mental illness believe that their
  mental illness makes it difficult to understand salvation.

- 49 percent of pastors report that they rarely or never speak about
  acute mental illness to their church in sermons or large groups.

- 23 percent of pastors have personally struggled with mental illness.[4]

Depression in American Christians is a real problem, and stigma is a
significant barrier to seeking and receiving effective treatment. Christians
with depression often are fearful of secular resources, and they don't know
where to turn. And sometimes they wait too long.

Pastors may not be aware that members of their congregation might
be waiting for them to proactively grant them permission to seek effective

3. Wesselmann et al., "Religious Beliefs," 165–68; Peteet, "Religiously Reinforced,"
846–48; Hankerson et al., "Ministers' Perceptions," 685–86.

4. Pingleton et al., "Mental Illness and Christian Faith," 5–8.

mental health care. Being silent on the topic of depression intensifies stigma, so at least a portion of each congregation needs the clergy to actively address the topic of depression and encourage professional treatment.

The Time to Get Help and Help Others Is Now

I want you to know that depression is treatable, and the sooner you tackle it, the better the outcome.[5] Throughout my over-twenty-year career in psychiatry, I have personally treated thousands of children and adults for a variety of psychiatric conditions, and I have helped hundreds of Christians. One pattern that I have seen repeatedly is that Christians often wait far too long before they seek effective help. They walk a long time through the darkest valley and can't find the path out. They experience unJoy. I can tell you that depression affects Christians and non-Christians alike.

I ask each new patient about their spirituality. One depressed teenage girl named Maria responded, "I'm a Christian." Her face then lit up like a ray of sunshine and she added, "I'm a child of God." She expressed her conviction so powerfully in that moment that the atmosphere in the room felt temporarily electrified. However, not long afterward, she looked sad again. With effective psychiatric care and counseling, her depression and suicidal thoughts improved substantially over the following weeks and months, and the smile on her face became more natural and frequent as her mood returned to its normal baseline.

This Is Not a Self-Help Book—It Is a Get-Help Book

This book is written by me, a Christian friend and physician who knows a lot about depression, to any Christian—you or someone you love—to let you know that depression is not your fault, and it is treatable.

From today forward, I strongly encourage you to give yourself full permission to seek help for depression.

There are many effective treatments for depression. When you think you might have depression, you need to start by determining if you have it, bringing your request for healing to God through prayer, making a decision to pursue effective treatment, and connecting with experts who know what they are doing.

5. Kraus et al., "Prognosis and Improved Outcomes," 1–8.

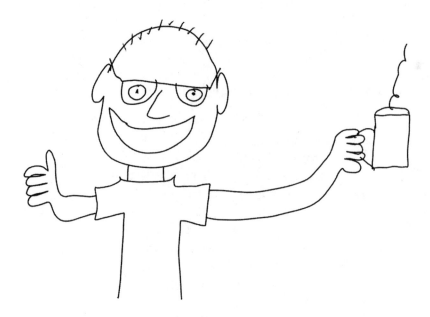

This is me encouraging you.

It takes courage to acknowledge that you are dealing with depression, especially if you fear that others won't understand or might negatively judge you. If you have depression, it is not because you are weak, lazy, sinful, or stupid. Depression is a medical condition no different from asthma, diabetes, or cancer, and like other medical conditions, it can improve with the right treatment. This book is about identifying your depression and saying, "I actually have depression and I have decided to do something effective about it," or "I know someone with depression and will share with them what I have learned." You will find enough information and encouragement in this book to get started. There are many ways to achieve full freedom from depression.

How to Read This Book and What You Will Find in the Chapters

Each chapter starts with a spiritual truth from the Bible. For each topic, I have included medical data from research and common-sense conclusions that can be drawn from the information. I have included interesting stories from my personal life, life in the church, and medical practice, and I explain real solutions that work.

This book contains twelve short chapters, which are grouped into three sections: I. Depression Is a Problem, and Emotional Pain Is Real; II. Solutions: Dealing with Depression as a Christian; III. The Journey to Health: Getting Better, Staying Better, and Helping Others.

At the end of each chapter, I have included questions for reflection for individuals and small groups. The goal of having you look through and answer the questions is to make the reading experience more interactive, to actively share your thoughts, and to draw your attention back to each chapter to help you remember the information.

To minimize the repetition of ideas, this book is organized to be read sequentially. Although you can skip around to read the chapters you are most interested in, you will have the best context for the ideas presented if you read the chapters in order.

Encouragement to Get Help and Be a Help to Others

Depression is treatable. It's time to do something about it! There are many ideas in this book for Christians with depression and for the clergy, family members, friends, and church members who love them. I recommend that you read this entire book and take immediate action to either effectively deal with your own depression or help others who you know are in need. If you are helping someone who has depression, please share this book with them. We can address depression and stigma in the church and share with our communities not just our support to them in their time of need but also the life-changing message of Jesus Christ.

Reflection

- Read Psalm 25:15–17. Do you believe this psalm applies to people suffering from depression? Why or why not?

- What is your reaction to the estimated number of Christians with depression? Do you believe the number, or does it seem too high or too low? Why?

- What is your reaction to the psychiatric nurse guessing that the young Christian woman who suffered for years before seeking help was Baptist? How might a person's Christian denomination influence stigma?

- Do you believe the medical data that Christians are at increased risk for stigma? Why or why not? What examples have you seen of mental health stigma among Christians? Why do you think that someone might hide their depression from others in the church? Do you believe that some Christians wait too long to get help, or do you think that people are too quick to label their problems as depression?

- Are there any other thoughts or memories that the introduction stirred up for you? Is there anything you wish you could share but don't feel comfortable sharing with people you know? Would sharing it with a professional who has sworn to maintain confidentiality make it easier to share?

- Are there any steps that you plan to take as a result of reading the introduction (for example, continue reading, get help for your depression, share this book with a friend)?

I

Depression Is a Problem, and Emotional Pain Is Real

1

Spiritual Battles, Sadness, Depression, Anxiety, or Boredom?

The Lord is close to the brokenhearted and saves
those who are crushed in spirit. (Psalm 34:18)

Depression and Its Relationship with Sadness

I HOPE THAT YOU'LL agree with me that sadness is a normal human emotion. Even Jesus wept (John 11:35). He is familiar with every aspect of your suffering as a "man of sorrows" (Isaiah 53:3).

And sadness is understandable in many situations. It's hard to know even where to start if you were to list how many situations there are in life that could understandably cause sadness. Grief over the loss of a loved one, loss of a job, or not having enough money are just a few of the common reasons to feel down. Sadness can occur over a disappointment with your kids, your spouse, or politics.

Depression and sadness are related but not the same thing. When I refer to depression, I'm talking about sadness at a whole different level. Depression means being stuck in sadness that might last hours, days, weeks, or months and occurs with other problems such as:

- Loss of enjoyment in pleasurable activities.
- Low motivation and energy.
- Crying spells.
- Appetite changes.
- Anxiety.
- Feelings of hopelessness, helplessness, or worthlessness.
- Sleep changes.
- Thoughts about killing yourself or wishing or praying for death or a fatal illness.

If that pattern lasts for two weeks or more and interferes with your ability to function well at home, work, or school, then the presence of depression is highly likely, and you should do something effective about it. If you think you might have depression, you can find the PHQ-9 depression screening tool in the "Resources" section at the back of this book to screen yourself for depression in a standardized way.

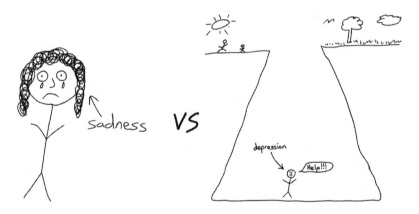

Sadness versus being stuck in the pit of depression.

I helped one of my older Christian relatives—I'll call him Jeff—get free from the depression he had suffered from for *seventy years*. Can you imagine being depressed for seventy years and then finally finding relief? After Jeff was free of depression, he said, "You have *no idea* what it feels like to *not* be depressed!"

Depression and Its Relationship with Anger

There are variations on depression that some people don't think about. For example, persistent anger or irritability—instead of sadness—along with the symptoms listed above could be depression. I've treated many patients who primarily wanted help for their anger and were surprised to learn that they actually had depression.

This is especially true for kids. Kids with depression often present as being extremely irritable rather than sad when they are depressed. And it can be complicated to sort out. Irritability in teenagers is part of their job description! It often takes professional expertise to sort out simply cranky teens from those with depression.

Depression Is Not Caused by Just One Thing

There are myths that depression is caused by just one thing, such as sin, laziness, or weakness, and some people think that the entire construct of depression is made up. I can tell you that these myths are simply not true. Alternatively, some people believe it is a certainty that you will become depressed if you experience stressful life events, such as cancer, the death of a spouse or child, bankruptcy, or divorce. That also is not true.

While negative life events can eventually result in depression, many other factors can contribute to its onset. Common risk factors include chronic pain, a past episode of depression, a serious medical condition, a traumatic event, active substance abuse, or a family history of depression.

Many biological factors contribute to depression, and researchers have continued to look for a single cause, such as neurotransmitters, hormones, or genetics, and they have come up short in finding a single unifying explanation as to what causes major depression. Neuroscience research has made some progress, which I'll talk about more in the next chapter, but it has a long way to go.

How Do Spiritual Battles Play a Role in Depression?

Christians with depression sometimes have spiritual battles as they wonder why bad things such as depression happen. Bad things can happen to strong Christians. Depression is one of those things. Sometimes people have the idea that if depression could be related to spiritual warfare, they should pray and wait. I can understand this reasoning, but I want to walk you through an idea.

Imagine that you were experiencing spiritual attacks that resulted in a broken bone or heart attack. How would you approach that? Would you (A) pray and wait, or (B) pray and seek medical care? Most Christians I know would choose option B; however, many Christians who have severe depression choose option A. Medical research clearly shows that the faster you get help for your depression, the better the outcome.[1] In the same way that I would encourage you to get immediate help for a heart attack or broken bone, I believe Christians with depression should seek help immediately.

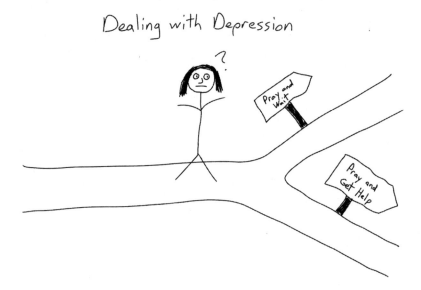

Have you heard the story of the Christian and the flood?

It's raining hard and a Christian who is at home watching the local meteorologist predict flooding hears someone pounding on the front door. A National Guardsman has a truck parked outside and says that floodwaters are rising, and he is here to take him to safety.

The Christian replies, "You can go. I have prayed to the Lord, and he will save me."

The Guardsman leaves. Not long afterward, water starts coming through the front door, so the Christian moves to the second floor of the house. Then a sheriff in a boat comes to the house.

1. Kraus et al., "Prognosis and Improved Outcomes," 1–8.

The sheriff says that the floodwaters are rising, and he is here to take him to safety.

The Christian replies, "You can go. I have prayed to the Lord, and he will save me."

The sheriff leaves. Not long afterward, the Christian is forced to climb onto the roof because of the rising water levels. Then a helicopter comes flying in through the storm and hovers over the house. The pilot shouts down for the Christian to grab the rope, as he is here to take him to safety.

The Christian shouts back, "You can go. I have prayed to the Lord, and he will save me."

The pilot leaves. Not long afterward, the Christian drowns in the flood. Then he wakes up in heaven. When he stands before God, he asks, "God, why didn't you save me?"

God replies, "What are you talking about? I sent you the truck, the boat, and the helicopter!"

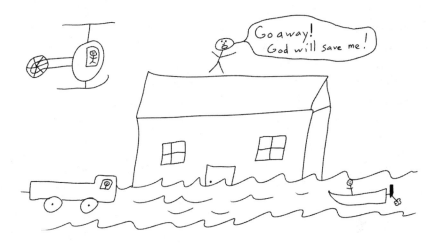

I understand that it can be confusing whether we should pray and wait or pray and seek medical care. I want to encourage you to choose option B. In the same way that God has provided cancer doctors for cancer, he has provided psychiatrists and counselors for depression. I strongly believe that Christians with depression need to use the help that God has provided.

Sin and Depression

Can sin lead to the onset of depression? Absolutely. However, sin is *not* the cause of most or all depressive episodes. Consider the following:

- All people sin, and most do not experience depression.
- Many people have no specific, repetitive, unconfessed sins, yet they develop depression.
- Some people develop depression after willfully sinning against God, yet after repenting and receiving forgiveness, the depression remains.

I strongly encourage all Christians to pray amid their depression. Depression itself can lead to spiritual confusion, so time in prayer will bring you closer to God during this difficult time in your life. Also, the enemy wants nothing more than to confuse you, separate you from God, and destroy you. If you believe that sin has contributed to the onset or continuation of your depression, then please pray to receive forgiveness and make a commitment to God to change your behavior. If your depression does not immediately lift and stay gone, then please seek professional help quickly. If you have done the above and some unhelpful person maintains that your depression is evidence that sin is the cause, please ignore that person and instead listen to people who are not eager to condemn you.

Depression and Its Relationship with Anxiety

Anxiety has been referred to in psychiatry as the Great Masquerader. Whether you want to call it stress, worry, fear, or nervousness, anxiety can be very tricky. At its extreme, it can fool people into thinking they are having a heart attack, seizure, or blindness. Anxiety can also contribute to or result in many different severe physical symptoms, such as abdominal pain, headaches/migraines, or other emotional problems such as depression.

Many people experience anxiety long before they become depressed. The anxiety continues to build and chip away at their physical and emotional reserves until they slip into depression. Among the patients I have worked with, many have expressed a strong belief that if their anxiety just went away, they would have no depression at all, and many of them might be correct. However, just as many people with depression have told me that they didn't have any anxiety until the start of their depression.

The reality is that depression and anxiety often go hand in hand. Anxiety can sometimes look a lot like depression. To make sure you are not confusing depression with stress and anxiety, you can complete the GAD-7 anxiety screening tool (found in the "Resources" section) and compare it to your PHQ-9 score. If your GAD-7 score is high but your PHQ-9 score is low, then maybe anxiety is the bigger problem for you.

When people become severely depressed, sometimes their anxiety goes down artificially. It's as though they have become so depressed and numb that the things that normally make them anxious no longer matter. At this point in their lives, anxiety is not a concern; however, it can become a huge concern once their depression starts to improve. Once depression improves, people start to *feel* again, and their old anxiety can resurface in a major way. It's important to know that as depression improves anxiety can worsen. In a way, it's a good problem to have, and if you know it might happen, you can prepare to effectively deal with it.

Depression and Its Relationship with Burnout

"Burnout" is not actually an official medical diagnosis. The condition was first described in the 1970s by a psychologist, Dr. Herbert Freudenberger.[2] He used the term "burnout" to conceptualize the state of severe exhaustion and stress that medical professionals experienced when sacrificing themselves in their professional roles for others. Common consequences of burnout include exhaustion, alienation, and reduced work performance. Burnout has taken on different meanings over time. More recently, it has become a safe way for people, especially medical professionals, to talk about a mixture of anxiety and depression from overload at work. There is less stigma in using the term "burnout" than the term "depression." "Burnout" is now the term doctors often use when they think they have depression or are headed toward depression.

Can Kids Really Get Depression?

Yes. The research is clear that 50 percent of lifetime mental illness starts by age fourteen and 75 percent of lifetime mental illness starts by age

---

2. Heinemann and Heinemann, "Burnout," 2–3.

twenty-four.[3] The difficult reality is that mental illness is primarily an illness of youth and can follow us into adulthood. When kids are struggling with mental illness, we need to get them help fast!

Depression in youth is not just a problem of today's generation. Do you remember Jeff from earlier in the chapter? He first experienced depression in the 1940s! At age *four*, he was so depressed that he asked his mother, calmly and seriously, to please kill him. It wasn't that there was no mental illness in the past, it was just that there was even more stigma and there were hardly any treatment options. Today, we have dozens of therapy approaches (chapter 7), antidepressant medications (chapter 8), and other powerful treatments for depression (chapters 9 and 10).

It is also important to note that chronic boredom in kids is a common precursor to sadness. Bored kids are frequently sad, and if this pattern lasts long enough, it can convert into depression.

Emotional Pain Is Real

Emotional pain is no less real than physical pain. What makes emotional pain even more challenging is that it can be harder to understand than physical pain. If you slam your hand in a door, you know why your hand hurts. Emotional pain is just as intense as—and sometimes more than—physical pain, but often you cannot identify the source.

That is one of the reasons why some people cope with their emotional pain in an unhealthy way by injuring themselves. Physical pain is easier to grasp and understand than emotional pain. And people do many things to try to cope with, avoid, or cover their emotional pain, such as abusing substances, overeating, hurting themselves physically, or engaging in out-of-control spending.

Other Types of Depression

While major depressive disorder is the most common type of depression, it also makes sense to consider other conditions that involve depression. In the same way that a person can have a massive swing *down* in their mood, they can have a massive swing *up* if they have a condition like bipolar I, bipolar II, or cyclothymia. If you have depressive symptoms, it is critical that

3. Kessler et al., "Lifetime Prevalence," 595–99.

you also be assessed for a bipolar-related illness, as different medications work for people with a bipolar illness.

This was true for my relative Jeff. He struggled with severe depression and suicidality since age four. In his lifetime, he had seen over a dozen psychiatrists. He had tried over a dozen antidepressant medications, electroconvulsive therapy (ECT), psychotherapy, and intense exercise, and had spent up to ten thousand dollars each year on vitamins. So, when he asked me for help, I was not surprised to hear that he hated modern medicine and psychiatrists (except for me, he assured me). Something that interfered with a correct diagnosis was that he could not provide me with the history I needed in order to understand what his illness was.

As a psychiatrist, I frequently need to hear from not just the patient but also from family members and other people in the person's life to get enough information to be confident in a diagnosis. I asked if I could speak with his wife to see what she observed. It turned out that Jeff did not have major depression. All of the medications he previously was prescribed either didn't help or caused his depression to worsen. Why? Because of the following equation: *wrong diagnosis = wrong treatment*. He had bipolar II disorder, which is similar to severe recurrent depression (it mostly manifests as sadness and anger), but it is distinctly different from major depression, especially regarding which medications work and which do not. I encouraged his primary care doctor to start him on a medication that is effective for bipolar II disorder. Thankfully, Jeff tolerated the medication well and reached remission of his depression for the first time in his life after *seventy years* of suffering.

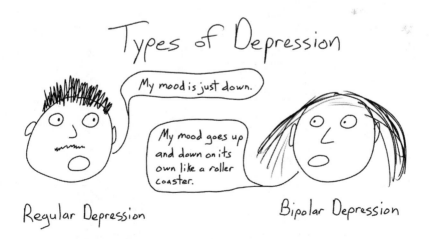

How Do You Screen for Bipolar Disorder?

Accurately distinguishing regular depression from bipolar disorder is one of the biggest challenges in psychiatry. However, if you have depression, it is important to spend the time to be thorough and assess for bipolar disorder. If you filled out the PHQ-9 in the "Resources" section, then it makes sense also for you to complete the MDQ bipolar screening tool (also in the "Resources" section). When I'm talking to patients, I might screen for bipolar by saying:

> I'm wondering if you have ever experienced something that almost felt like the exact opposite of depression, several symptoms that all occur together at the same time and last for two to five days or longer. Have you ever had symptoms of decreased need for sleep (you had less sleep and yet you were more energized), racing thoughts (not just anxious thoughts that are spinning in circles but feeling like you're thinking in fast-forward), an extra happy mood, a very elevated sex drive (or being especially physically affectionate towards others), and a feeling of invincibility (almost as though you have superpowers, a million dollars in the bank, or are completely convinced that something amazing is going to happen in your life)?

I might follow this questioning up with, "Have you ever experienced a very weird mood, such as feeling incredibly happy and incredibly sad at the exact same time for hours or days at a time?" or "Have you been experiencing extremely high moods followed by extremely sad moods with absolutely no warning or trigger between the mood switches?"

My experience is that people who say the above descriptions resonate strongly with them tend to score high on the MDQ in the "Resources" section. People with bipolar disorder should work with a skilled psychiatrist, as regular depression treatments can result in bigger mood swings and overall worsened mood. While primary care can be a good place for people with major depression to start, primary care physicians often struggle to provide the level of care needed for both mood stability and freedom from depressive symptoms for people with bipolar disorder.

Finding Direction in Treatment

Getting help for depression involves an accurate diagnosis, a commitment to taking action quickly, and working with a skilled professional. Do you believe that depression exists and that emotional pain is real? I strongly do. I can also tell you that spiritual battles are not the only explanation for depression. People of all ages, including children, can experience depression. While life stresses can result in normal sadness, it is important to determine if you have depression, especially if you are sad or mad often. If you have depression, make a point to get an assessment for bipolar disorder and make sure that your psychiatrist and therapist are paying attention to the role that anxiety is playing in your mood. The right diagnosis will help you get the right treatment so you can achieve freedom from depression and thrive like God intends you to.

Reflection

- Read Psalm 34, especially taking note of verse 18. How do you believe this verse applies to people going through depression? What do you think it means that God is "close" to the brokenhearted?

- What differences do you see between sadness and depression?

- Do you believe that a person can be experiencing spiritual battles and an episode of depression at the same time?

- What do you see in terms of the interplay of stress/anxiety and depression among the people you know?

- What do you think about the statistics that show that mental health problems begin early in life?

- Do you believe that life circumstances that cause understandable sadness can lead to full-on depression? Why or why not?

- What is your reaction to the story of Jeff, who had depression for seventy years and whose depression was misdiagnosed and mistreated for decades until he got effective help?

- What do you think about the assertion that emotional pain is real pain?

- If you thought you or a loved one had depression, how would you go about dealing with it?

- Are there any steps that you plan to take as a result of reading this chapter (for example, sharing the depression quizzes with others, taking the quizzes yourself, or sharing your concerns with a trusted loved one or professional)?

2

Stigma Can Lead to Guilt, Shame, and Doubt

I sought the Lord, and he answered me; he delivered me
from all my fears. Those who look to him are radiant; their
faces are never covered with shame. (Psalm 34:4–5)

What Are the Negative Effects of Stigma?

MENTAL HEALTH STIGMA CAN make people feel alone even when they are surrounded by people who love them. In addition to feelings of isolation, stigma can fuel other negative emotions, such as shame, guilt, and doubt. Both the symptoms of depression and the stigma surrounding it can lead people to develop a sense that something is inherently wrong with them or that they are too weak or lazy to just "snap out of" their depression.

Mental health stigma can lead people to feel trapped in inaction, which results in suffering for far too long. It is understandable how people can become so stuck or ambivalent about doing something about their depression. They might fear that they will make the wrong choices, that the solutions will fail, or that they will be judged by others on how they choose to get help.

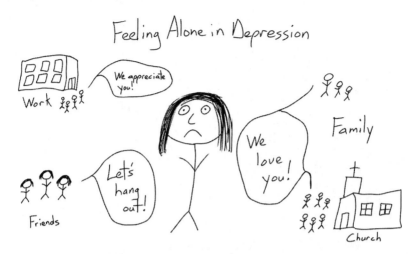

When dealing with depression, it is common to feel isolated and alone even when you are around others who are encouraging.

There are seven million Christians who have major depression every year, and a significant portion of them work to keep it a secret. If you experience depression, I want you to know that there is no cause for shame. I hope to show you through logic and medical research why the myths surrounding stigma just aren't true. Also, I want to share with you some steps that you can take to get help even if you still believe the stigma myths or if you think that the medical condition of depression is an artificial construct. Essentially, my hope is to convince you to get effective help for yourself or others with depression even if you find yourself disagreeing with me in some way.

A Medical Reason to Have No Guilt or Shame about Depression

Check out the drawing below.

What this diagram from medical research shows is that there is different brain activity in a depressed brain compared to a non-depressed brain.[1] Brain activity is clearly different in people with depression!

---

1. Williams, "Precision Psychiatry," 473–75.

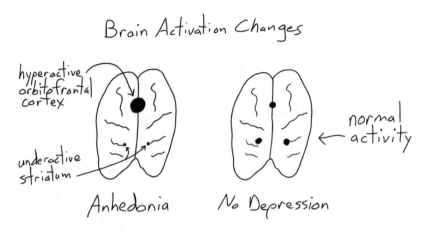

This is my attempt at drawing a cross-section of the human brain. Medical research clearly shows a different brain activation pattern with anhedonia (unJoy) compared to a person without depression.

It is clear that there is a specific, abnormal brain activation pattern that is present in people who have anhedonia, which is a prominent feature of major depression, and absent in those who do not. Anhedonia is the inability to experience pleasure or joy in life. If you had to boil down major depression to a single symptom, it would be "anhedonia," or what I call "unJoy." Many other symptoms can go along with mood disorders, but anhedonia is one of the most definitive symptoms of depression.

In my clinical practice, I frequently hear from patients, "I shouldn't be depressed. I have a good life. If my friends or coworkers knew I was depressed, they wouldn't understand or they would be mad at me. They think I have it made. So, why don't I feel that way?" The diagram above helps to explain why. People with depression frequently and repeatedly blame themselves for their depression. I don't believe it makes sense to blame yourself for abnormal brain activity. Do you? Do you know anyone who can control their brain activity? The diagram above is scientific research that helps to answer the question, "Why do I feel depressed when my life is good?"

My response to these patients is, "You are right. Your life is good. Your depression is due to your brain activity being stuck out of balance and the regions of your brain not communicating correctly. That's why you feel depressed when everything around you is good."

I help many people with treatment-resistant depression through a medical intervention called transcranial magnetic stimulation (TMS) therapy (which I'll discuss further in chapter 9). When I explain to people what is going on in their brain when they have depression and how the treatment works—essentially to reverse these abnormalities—and that the treatment has excellent odds of success, their entire demeanor changes. You can see the weight they've been carrying around immediately start to lift. They realize there is a biological explanation for why they feel so depressed when their lives are good, and their self-blame starts to drop. People start to feel hope. It motivates them to work with mental health professionals to get rid of their depression as quickly as possible.

There Are Medical Diseases That Cause and Mimic Depression

People are so different when it comes to medical care. Some people are quick to seek medical help, and others only go to a doctor in dire situations. Even if you avoid doctors like the plague, you need to see one if you suspect you have depression. Here is the reason: it might be due to a physical illness. If a medical condition was causing or worsening your depression, wouldn't you want to know? Wouldn't your loved ones want you to get medical care?

Many medical conditions can cause or mimic depression. Some of these include:

- Thyroid abnormality.
- Low vitamin D.
- Iron deficiency anemia.
- Low vitamin B12.
- Autoimmune disorders.
- Infectious diseases.
- Medication side effects.
- Chronic pain.
- Obstructive sleep apnea.
- Fibromyalgia and chronic fatigue syndrome.

In my medical practice, I have found all of the above medical conditions as a cause of depression or worsening depressive symptoms.

Labels under Which You Can Receive Care That May Be Less Stigmatizing

Some people would never accept a label of depression, and that keeps them from pursuing treatment. There are many reasons why people do not want to have a formal mental health diagnosis. They ask, "Can't I just get help for my anger? Just put 'anger' down as the diagnosis on the chart. Okay, Doc?"

While for seventy years there was a requirement that a person had to be labeled with a formal mental health diagnosis to get their health insurance companies to cover their treatments, on October 1, 2018, the United States government approved the use of some new diagnosis codes for mental health concerns that are not officially recognized as illnesses by the field of psychiatry. Here is a list of some of them (with ICD-10-CM codes):[2]

- Nervousness (R45.0).

- Restlessness and agitation (R45.1).

- Unhappiness (R45.2).

- Demoralization and apathy (R45.3).

- Anger and irritability (R45.4).

- Hostility (R45.5).

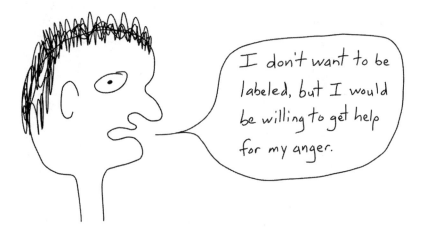

2. National Center for Health Statistics, "ICD-10-CM."

Your health insurance might cover mental health treatment for a concern/symptom rather than a psychiatric diagnostic label. I would guess that most primary care physicians and psychiatrists are unaware of this change in the diagnosis codes. If this issue is important to you, one of the first things you can do is educate your doctor about the above options for diagnoses and inform them that you want treatment for your primary concern, not for a different diagnostic label that you find stigmatizing.

Getting Help for Yourself Because You Care about Others

I have seen many people—parents and spouses in particular—make heroic sacrifices because of their love for others. These Christians often strongly embody Jesus's command, "Love your neighbor as yourself" (Matthew 22:39). They will work crazy hours and deny themselves even small rewards to give what they have—their time, talents, and finances—to others rather than themselves. Their generosity and altruism can tremendously benefit others but leave them feeling depleted. They often are unwilling to take the time and the expense to deal with their own depression.

If you are one of these people, I have a message for you.

Put on your own oxygen mask first.

If you have ever flown on a commercial airline, you have heard that announcement about what to do if the oxygen masks drop down from the ceiling. You are instructed to put your own mask on before helping others. The message is clear: you cannot help others if you have already passed out. Well, the same is true if you have depression. If you allow your depression to worsen to the point that you are having trouble caring for yourself, how on earth will you be able to help others? The truth is that you won't. The very people you support and who rely on you will be scrambling to figure out how to help *you*.

I want you to know that you are worth the time and the money that it takes to get free from depression as quickly as possible. It is a good investment. If you are used to always sacrificing your needs for others, you will need to make your mental health a priority.

And if you are a pastor or Christian leader reading this, this means you, too. Actively and effectively taking care of your mental health is proof of your fitness for ministry. Take care of yourself! You cannot pour from an empty cup.

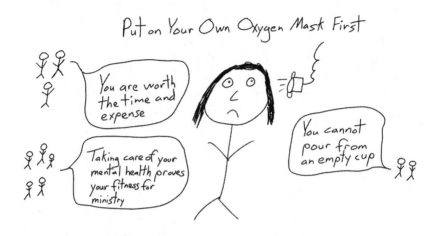

Every Church Community Can Address Mental Health Stigma

Substantial mental health stigma exists in Christian communities. According to research,[3] 49 percent of pastors report that they rarely or never speak about acute mental illness to their church in sermons or large groups. We can address mental health stigma in Christianity and help our Christian brothers and sisters with depression. There are several steps that churches can take to reduce stigma. At my own church, our pastor and other leaders have addressed mental health stigma as part of a natural expression of our Christian faith. At our church, we have:

- Participated in and cleaned up a local park after the annual NAMI Walk, which is an event to decrease mental health stigma led by the Montana chapter of the National Alliance on Mental Illness.

- Had sermon series on wrestling with mental illness as a Christian.

- Held training on suicide prevention and invited others in our community to attend.

- Had a "Conversation at the Well" series in which the pastor interviewed church members during a worship service about their faith and Christian walk. My wife and I participated on separate Sundays. We shared how we felt called to specialize in psychiatry following

---

3. Pingleton et al., "Mental Illness and Christian Faith," 5–8.

medical school and how our faith impacts our medical practice. Other church members shared their personal struggles, and several shared their experiences with depression.

Having openly addressed mental health issues and actively supported mental health organizations in our community, our church members have felt more comfortable sharing struggles with depression with no more stigma than discussing having diabetes or asthma. There are other approaches that churches can use to address mental health stigma, including:

- Small group studies on depression and faith.
- Clear communication from the pastor and leadership that depression and emotional pain are real.
- Eliminating the unhelpful and incorrect message that most depression is caused by undiscovered or undisclosed sin. Yes, it is always important to pray. However, it also is important to get a depressed person to a highly competent professional. Clinical depression treatments work effectively for Christians with depression.
- Direct encouragement by ministry leaders and counselors that having depression is not a person's fault, but it is their responsibility to take real steps to deal with it.
- Sharing books for the layperson with depression that meet the definition of "bibliotherapy" (books shown by research to decrease depression and/or suicide risk).
- Decreasing the expectation that a Christian can work only with a self-identified Christian counselor or psychiatrist.

Getting Stigma Out of Your Way

While stigma can block Christians from quickly dealing with their depression, there are ways of addressing the stigma head on. One of the first steps is to acknowledge that stigma exists and might be present in your life so it is not lingering and undermining your efforts. The next step is to actively diminish self-blame by recognizing that there are brain signaling and activation changes that occur in depression and that some medical conditions cause and worsen depression. If you have a fear or concern about receiving a formal psychiatric diagnosis, there are methods of obtaining quality mental health care without those labels. If you have depression, then you need and deserve help. If you routinely sacrifice your needs for the needs of others, it is critical that you get rid of your depression so you will be able to more effectively help others.

Reflection

- Read Psalm 34, focusing especially on verses 4–5. Do you believe these verses apply to people fearful of stigma? Why?

- How do you think Christians encounter mental health stigma?

- Would you be concerned about what others thought of you if they knew you had depression? What would concern you the most?

- What do you think of the brain activation changes in depression?

- If you had depression, would you consider meeting with your doctor to see if it was caused by another medical condition? If not, why?

- If you had depression, would you be more likely to get help in order to feel better yourself, or because others are counting on you?

- If you went to your doctor for depression, would you rather have a depression diagnosis or something else, such as "unhappiness," "demoralization and apathy," or "anger and irritability?"

- Are there any steps that you plan to take as a result of reading this chapter (for example, sharing some of these ideas with others or scheduling to see your doctor)?

3

You Can Change Negative Thoughts to Improve Your Depression

Why, my soul, are you downcast? Why so disturbed
within me? Put your hope in God, for I will yet praise
him, my Savior and my God. (Psalm 42:5)

Thoughts Can Cause Emotions

Do you believe that? Because it's true. Most of our emotions are preceded by a thought or an event. The thought, "I'm going to get a raise!" will increase your feelings of happiness at work a lot more than the thought, "I'm going to get fired!"

One of the challenges for people with depression is that they tend to have a lot of negative thoughts. These thoughts may occur automatically and often are so unbalanced that they aren't true, yet the depressed person believes them.

There is hope. You might not believe me, so you'll have to trust me on this one: *you can actually change your thoughts.* This might sound impossible or dangerous, but it is possible, and I'm not talking about brainwashing. What I'm talking about is recognizing unbalanced thoughts as untrue and getting to a place where you can quickly conquer negative thoughts and take control of your emotions.

Unbalanced or Untrue Thoughts Can Amplify Our Emotions

Unbalanced thoughts can trigger huge emotional reactions. Ultimately, the reason for this overreaction in our emotions is because the thought is simply not true. We might believe the thought, "I'm a failure," triggering feelings of despair and sadness. However, that thought is not true. Having struggled at one thing or many things does not make a person a failure. Consider this: leaders who have been identified as successful have had far more failures cumulatively than the average person. They just considered their failed attempts to be lessons learned and temporary setbacks as they plowed forward.

It's believing the lie that gives such power and emotional control to a thought. For some people, their negative thoughts are relatively automatic. These thoughts just spring into their minds over and over. While it can be a challenge to fix these thoughts on your own, working with a professional skilled in cognitive behavioral therapy (CBT is discussed in more detail in chapter 7) can help you deal with negative automatic thoughts so effectively that you can counter the automatic thoughts *automatically* and stay in control of your emotions.

Thought Balancing

Thought balancing is a process of looking at facts or data that support or refute negative thoughts. As you list all of the ways that a thought is accurate and inaccurate, you will be able to develop a new, true thought to counter or replace the untrue, negative thought. The more accurate and powerful the new thought is, the better you will be able to eliminate the unbalanced one. There are several benefits to doing this. One is that the more you work on balancing your thoughts, the more you will be able to quickly replace negative thoughts. Another benefit is that you will not need to be in therapy forever because, in a way, you will have learned how to be your own therapist. The ultimate benefit of practicing thought balancing is that you will simply become a happier person.

The process of balancing your thoughts is often called cognitive reframing. Here is a situation from my life that we can use as an example of how cognitive reframing works: I was driving to work in dense traffic and a guy in a muddy, jacked-up pickup in the lane next to me swerved into my lane right in front of me. I had to hit my brakes and swerve, and I honked my car horn. The guy just kept speeding down the road! I thought, "He thinks he owns the road! He tried to kill me!" I felt really angry, and my anger lingered, ruining my entire morning.

I had a chance to think through the situation at lunchtime. When I considered alternative thoughts to my initial one, my emotions changed. I first considered the thought, "That man was not trying to murder me," which was true and helped my anger a little. I then considered the thought, "His truck is higher than my car, so he might not have seen me." That helped my anger a bit more. Then I took my thinking a step further by considering, "He could have been rushing somewhere important, like the hospital, or maybe someone he cares about—like a child—is in trouble and he's going to help them." With those final thoughts, my anger vanished. Can you see how powerful thoughts are and how cognitive reframing can rapidly change your emotions?

Intrusive Thoughts

Intrusive thoughts are unwanted, negative thoughts that are not in alignment with your values. Intrusive thoughts force their way into a person's awareness and feel like they come out of nowhere. These thoughts tend to freak people out. Examples of these types of thoughts would be thinking of killing yourself or someone else, harming a child, or having mental images of pornography.

I have helped many patients recognize and deal with their intrusive thoughts. They express enormous relief at knowing what the thoughts are and that they can deal with them. It starts with recognizing the thoughts as intrusive—essentially separate from your identity and values—and then "talking back" to the intrusive thoughts. Helpful methods for talking back to intrusive thoughts include saying:

- "That's just a thought."
- "Having a thought is different from intentionally dwelling on it."
- "I'm not that thought."
- "Oh. There's that old thought again."

You can use these methods to disarm intrusive thoughts and dismiss them from your mind because you know that they are not true, they are not you, and they do not represent you or your values.

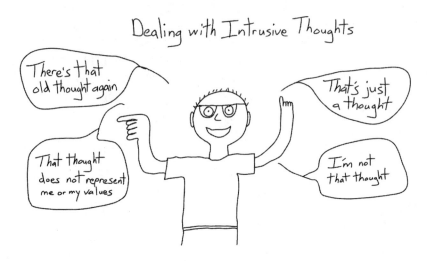

Dealing with Intrusive Thoughts

There's that old thought again

That's just a thought

That thought does not represent me or my values

I'm not that thought

hm

Using Biblical Affirmations to Counter Negative Thoughts

For people with depression, untrue thoughts can feel true. This is called emotional reasoning. If you feel guilty, you assume you must have done something wrong. If you feel hopeless, you just might start to believe that you are hopeless. Emotional reasoning can be incredibly confusing, especially if you do not have an effective strategy for combating it.

People with depression can find themselves dwelling on negative thoughts for hours at a time. Sometimes finding a positive, alternative thought just doesn't do it for them. I work with many patients who find that spending time meditating on affirming verses in the Bible is a welcome relief to negative thoughts. Given that negative, unbalanced thoughts are untrue, it is appropriate to counter them with biblical truths.

Emotional reasoning of, "I'm in such pain. There will never be any relief," can be replaced with:

> Praise be to the God and Father of our Lord Jesus Christ, the Father of compassion and the God of all comfort, who comforts us in all our troubles, so that we can comfort those in any trouble with the comfort we ourselves receive from God. (2 Corinthians 1:3–4)

Emotional reasoning of, "I don't feel God's presence. I don't think he hears my prayers," can be replaced with:

> *I love the Lord, for he heard my voice; he heard my cry for mercy. Because he turned his ear to me, I will call on him as long as I live. (Psalm 116:1–2)*

Emotional reasoning of, "My pain will never end," can be replaced with:

> *Your sun will never set again, and your moon will wane no more; the Lord will be your everlasting light, and your days of sorrow will end. (Isaiah 60:20)*

Emotional reasoning of, "I feel so defeated. Nothing can help me," can be replaced with:

> *God is our refuge and strength, an ever-present help in trouble. Therefore we will not fear, though the earth give way and the mountains fall into the heart of the sea. (Psalm 46:1–2)*

Emotional reasoning of, "I feel so alone. Nobody cares about me," can be replaced with:

> *He heals the brokenhearted and binds up their wounds. (Psalm 147:3)*

There are many other biblical affirmations that might resonate more powerfully with you. Use them. Meditate on encouraging passages from God's word rather than dwelling on repetitive, negative thoughts or relying on emotional reasoning.

Taking Action on Depression When It Interferes with Positive Memories

Have you ever noticed that a depressed person seems to forget the positive things in their lives? It's as though they have forgotten all their positive memories. There is a reason for this, and it is related to a biological process called state-dependent learning. People's minds record memories in the situational context that the event occurred. Everything gets recorded together: the place, the emotions, the people, the sights, the sounds, and the smells. Have you ever been transported to a powerful memory just by a certain smell? Your memory was tied to that smell.

Well, it's hard for people who are depressed to strongly remember positive memories because just as there is state-dependent learning there is a process called state-dependent recall. It is easier to remember details of a memory when you are back in that same situation. It is hard for depressed people to strongly remember positive memories when they are depressed. When the depression lifts, their ability to recall positive memories improves.

Is there anything you can do about that? Absolutely! If you have been around a severely depressed person, you might have noticed that a positive activity can lift their spirits at least temporarily. There is a strategy called behavioral activation (which I'll talk more about in chapter 6) that involves planning throughout each day multiple different activities that are in alignment with the person's values. Behavioral activation has been shown to exert a powerful, positive influence on depression.[1] This positive effect may be due to several factors. Behavioral activation activities can get a depressed person into a positive emotional state to access positive memories and remember a time when life was good. Additionally, these activities send powerful signals to the depressed brain to become more active and function in a non-depressed way.

Self-Absorption and Depression

I'm not sure if you have observed this, but sometimes people with depression exhibit an increase in self-centeredness. It's not their fault! Please understand that they are not doing this intentionally or using their depression as an excuse to get their way. It is due to something called depressive rumination (dwelling on negative thoughts). Check out the following diagram:

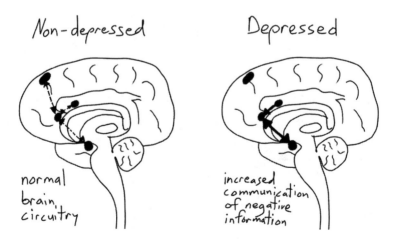

Non-depressed

Depressed

normal brain circuitry

increased communication of negative information

1. Mazzucchelli et al., "Behavioral Activation," 399–404.

This diagram conveys medical evidence that rumination is not something that depressed people wish upon themselves. There are changes in signaling or communication between the cognitive reasoning (frontal lobe) and emotional control (limbic system) regions of the brains of people with depression. One very interesting research finding is that there is increased signaling/communication along specific neural pathways that are responsible for providing information with *negative* content.[2] In other words, the diagram above shows that there is biological activity involved in depressive rumination, the mental process that can make depressed people seem selfish.

People with depression can become overly preoccupied with themselves and their needs. The constant chatter of their own thoughts can drown out their ability to hear and pay attention to others' needs. Rumination occurs commonly in depression. It's essentially what the brain does when it is trying to make sense of an upsetting situation or solve a difficult problem. Many depressed people have the incorrect belief that ruminative thoughts are helpful. Common ruminative thoughts include:

- "I never used to have this kind of trouble. Why can't I do what I used to do?"

- "What's causing this? What is stopping me from getting better?"

- "Other people don't have this problem, so why do I?"

While some people appeared selfish before they ever became depressed, the majority of people develop self-absorption due to worsening depression. This self-centeredness appears to be due to a tunnel-vision effect on a depressed person's thinking and awareness. And if a person actually was selfish and had trouble listening and connecting to others before the onset of their depression, the depression will worsen those traits.

There are ways of combating depressive rumination and how it manifests as self-absorption or selfishness. The first is the strategy of behavioral activation that was mentioned above. Research shows that behavioral activation is as effective as a full course of CBT, even though behavioral activation isn't confronting the unbalanced thoughts.[3] In a way, the actions and activities themselves in behavioral activation prove that the negative thoughts are untrue because the person is accomplishing and often enjoying activities their depressed mind told them were impossible.

2. Pizzagalli, "Frontocingulate Dysfunction," 191–93.
3. Gortner et al., "Cognitive-Behavioral," 379–80.

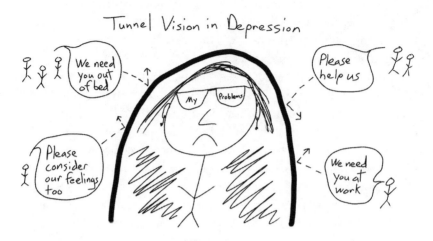

There also is a form of CBT called rumination-focused cognitive behavioral therapy (RFCBT), which relies on a combination of behavioral experiments, experiential exercises, and shifting from unconstructive rumination to constructive rumination.[4]

Using Mindfulness to Silence Negative Thoughts and Stop Beating Yourself Up

A final way to combat depressive rumination is through mindfulness strategies, which involve holding one's mental concentration on a different area of focus (not on the negative thought) and then practicing not criticizing yourself when your focus wavers. Research shows that mindfulness strategies can decrease depressive rumination.[5]

Many people have a powerful, out-of-control Inner Critic. The Inner Critic is not a hallucination, but rather is our own internal critical voice that tells us that we are lazy, stupid, ugly, greedy, selfish, and unworthy frauds. It robs us of confidence, joy, and satisfaction, and it often is not reality-based. The Inner Critic is one of the biggest drivers of feelings of insecurity. It can contribute to depression and also be fed by depression.

Our self-critical thoughts are a double-edged sword. They can motivate us, drive us to try harder through fear of failure, and push us to the limits of our abilities. While many people value being hard on themselves

4. Watkins et al., "Rumination-Focused," 317–18.

5. Ramel et al., "Mindfulness," 442–47.

and they may credit part or all of their success to it, the Inner Critic can fuel anxiety, depression, and hopelessness.

If you have a powerful Inner Critic, there is hope for positive change. Common statements from Inner Critics include:

- "You don't deserve what you have."
- "Someone is going to find out what a fraud you are."
- "You're so stupid."
- "What's wrong with you?"

You can combat the Inner Critic through mindfulness. This is a process of bringing your attention to one center of focus, thinking about one thing instead of allowing your mind to drift to other topics. By practicing mindfulness, you can learn to calm your mind. You can learn how to sharpen your focus and block out distracting and unhelpful thoughts, and in doing so you can practice not judging yourself so harshly. When you notice your mind has wandered, gently bring your awareness back to whatever you were originally focused on, being kind to yourself as you do so. Getting distracted happens to everyone. For more information on mindfulness exercises, you can access free articles and information at my website (lenlantz.com/unJoy).

The Inner Critic

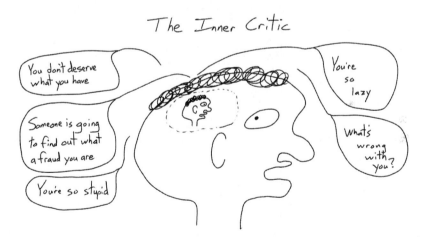

Mindfulness and some meditative practices can also center on verses of the Bible. Please know that I am *not* talking about transcendental meditation. Instead, I am referring to biblical meditation, an example being *lectio divina* (literally, "divine reading"), which is a form of biblical meditation originating in Catholicism. While it has been practiced for centuries and uses mindfulness strategies to dwell on God's word, there is concern about its practice in some Protestant denominations. If you don't feel comfortable with the practice of *lectio divina*, there are other ways to meditate on God's word using mindfulness strategies. The Bible is filled with positive references to meditating on God and his word (Psalm 19:14, Psalm 104:34, Psalm 119, Psalm 143:5–6, Psalm 145:5, Colossians 3:16).

J. I. Packer references meditating on God and his word in his classic book *Knowing God*: "Meditation is the activity of calling to mind, and thinking over, and dwelling on, and applying to oneself, the various things that one knows about the works and ways and purposes and promises of God. It is an activity of holy thought, consciously performed in the presence of God, under the eye of God, by the help of God, as a means of communion with God."[6]

It Is Possible to Improve Depression by Changing Negative Thoughts

You can dramatically improve your mood by changing your negative thoughts. There are many strategies for doing this, including thought balancing, cognitive reframing, distraction, positive activities that are in alignment with your values, formal psychotherapy, and meditative and mindful practices. What strategy would you feel the most comfortable starting? It is possible to silence self-critical thoughts and focus more on uplifting ones. Reviewing your options for intervention, selecting a solution that you like, and making a commitment to use that strategy to battle thinking errors is the place to start. Imagine the relief that you will feel when you prove to yourself that you can control your emotions as you more effectively control your thoughts.

Reflection

- Read Psalm 42. How does this psalm apply to negative thinking?
- Can you think of examples of thoughts causing emotions?

6. Packer, *Knowing God*, 18–19.

- Do you believe that unbalanced thoughts can lead to big emotional reactions? Why or why not?

- What do you think of the idea of changing your thoughts to change your emotions?

- Does knowing what an intrusive thought is help you in any way? If so, how?

- Have you ever used biblical affirmations in your life? What was your experience?

- What do you think about self-absorption and ruminative thoughts in depression?

- Do you think that meditation and mindfulness could be helpful practices to combat negative thoughts? Why or why not?

- Are there any steps that you plan to take as a result of reading this chapter (for example, writing down affirmation verses from the Bible, creating a schedule of behavioral activation activities, or developing the discipline of meditating on God and his word)?

4

Suicide, Self-Destructive Thoughts, and Heaven

*Let us hold unswervingly to the hope we profess, for
he who promised is faithful. (Hebrews 10:23)*

Suicide Is a Tough Problem for Everyone

MAKE NO MISTAKE—SUICIDE HURTS everybody, even psychiatrists. We try
not to show how sad and demoralized it makes us feel because family and
friends who are left behind are counting on us and need us in their time of
crisis, but losing a patient to suicide is an incredibly painful experience that
I have personally gone through. It's one of my reasons for writing this book.

From me to you: *If you are having suicidal thoughts, please connect
with a professional immediately.*

God put a conviction in my heart to do something about suicide in
Montana, which has one of the highest suicide rates in the nation. Starting
in the fall of 2012, I just couldn't shake the idea that if we had such high
suicide rates, there had to be *something*—something basic—that we could
do to prevent suicide. I attempted two approaches, not knowing if either
would move forward, and God brought both to fruition. My first effort was
to request passage of a state law creating the Montana Suicide Mortality

Review Team, which I chaired as we looked for patterns among all the suicides that occurred in Montana over a two-year period. Our findings helped shape the state's suicide prevention plan.

My second effort was to create the Montana Conference on Suicide Prevention, which I chaired and hosted for its first seven years. The goal of the conference was to bring together community members, clergy, law enforcement, state leaders, and mental health professionals all in one room to learn strategies for immediately preventing suicide. We trained thousands of people free of charge, and the annual conference is continuing to grow.

Did these efforts lower the suicide rate? Time will tell. I can tell you one thing, which is that I gave it my best shot and am trusting God with the results. I haven't stopped supporting suicide prevention and am continuing to participate in other ways to make a difference. And I have learned a few things along the way:

- Virtually everyone has been affected and hurt in some way by suicide.

- There are many passionate and strong opinions about what the best solutions are.

- More research on suicide prevention is desperately needed.

- Our suicide rates in the nation continue to rise.

- People contemplating suicide need realistic hope *and* immediate help.

God Has Called Christians to Perseverance, Not Suicide

Yearning for heaven is understandable. To a depressed person in pain—a person who feels like they are already dying—heaven is greatly desired. It's understandable for people in misery to want to be released from the present earth and the problems of life. You might not really grasp how desirable heaven is until you have viewed it through the eyes of the severely depressed Christian. While heaven is awesome, dying by suicide is not logical and it is not God's plan for us. God has not called Christians to suicide but to perseverance.

> But he said to me, "My grace is sufficient for you, for my power is made perfect in weakness." Therefore I will boast all the more gladly about my weaknesses, so that Christ's power may rest on me. That is why, for Christ's sake, I delight in weaknesses, in insults, in

hardships, in persecutions, in difficulties. For when I am weak, then I am strong. (2 Corinthians 12:9–10)

Suicide Is a Burden on Loved Ones

I'll talk more later on the thinking errors of suicidal people, but one issue that immediately needs to be addressed is the irrational idea that some suicidal people have that they are a burden on others. They think that by killing themselves, they will be less of a burden. That thought is false on many levels.

You are not a burden, but your suicide would be a burden.

Suicides have a destructive ripple effect. The pain of one person dying by suicide spreads outward, affecting the person's loved ones. The person's friends and relatives are left wondering, "What if?"

- "What if I could have been more encouraging?"

- "What if I had called or text messaged them when I thought of it?"

- "What if I could have done something to prevent their death?"

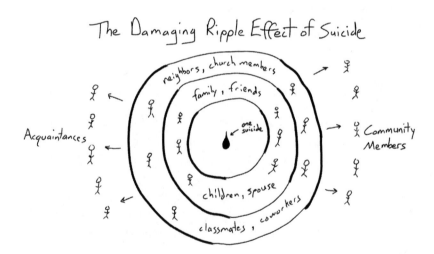

The Damaging Ripple Effect of Suicide

Many people are also unaware of the risk that suicide places on others. Research shows that children and teens whose parents die by suicide have a *three times higher risk* of dying by suicide themselves.[1] Also, if a person dies

1. Wilcox et al., "Parental Death," 518.

by suicide, it significantly increases the risk of suicide among other family and friends grieving the loss.[2] There also is a risk of contagion (copy-cat suicides), especially among youth.

Rather than decreasing the burden on others, when people die by suicide, they are essentially handing their bucket of pain to everyone who cares about them.

God Is Opposed to Suicide

God is opposed to suicide, as it would be breaking his commandments and forcing your will upon God. Theologians have wrestled with suicide and how it relates to the Christian walk. Some have pointed to the Ten Commandments as God's instruction against suicide because it is a form of self-murder.

> *You shall not murder. (Exodus 20:13)*

God also tells us that he has determined the length of our lives in advance. Who are we to presume to force God's hand or inform God how many days we will live?

> *Your eyes saw my unformed body; all the days ordained for me were written in your book before one of them came to be. (Psalm 139:16)*

Jesus taught that the second greatest commandment is to love our neighbors as ourselves. Suicide causes others to suffer and increases the risk of suicide of children and other loved ones who are left behind.

> *Jesus replied: "'Love the Lord your God with all your heart and with all your soul and with all your mind.' This is the first and greatest commandment. And the second is like it: 'Love your neighbor as yourself.'" (Matthew 22:37–39)*

The early Christian reformer John Calvin expressed his views on suicide. According to historian Jeffrey R. Watt, Calvin "categorically condemned it primarily because it was a rebellion against God, a refusal to submit to God's will."[3] The Christian writer and philosopher C. S. Lewis

---

2. Pitman et al., "Bereavement by Suicide," 4–8.

3. Watt, "Calvin on Suicide," 474.

also addressed the topic of suicide and ultimately concluded, "You must go on. That is one of the many reasons why suicide is out of the question."[4]

Suicide Is the Result of Thinking Errors

Medical experts maintain that suicide is the result of thinking errors. Depression expert Dr. David Burns—whose father, incidentally, was a Lutheran minister—really understands the thinking errors that occur in depression and states, "You are wrong in your belief that suicide is the only solution or the best solution to your problem. Let me repeat that. *You are wrong!* When you think that you are trapped and hopeless, your thinking is illogical, distorted, and skewed. No matter how thoroughly you have convinced yourself, and even if you get other people to agree with you, you are just plain *mistaken* in your belief that it is ever advisable to commit suicide because of depressive illness."[5]

I've shared with patients that I see depression as a liar. Depression can dramatically distort people's thinking so they believe the lies. Then, when the depressed person is vulnerable (feeling hopeless, overwhelmed, or intoxicated), all they can think about is dying, and they start to strongly believe the common *lies* of depression:

- "You'll always feel this way."
- "You'll never get better."
- "There is nothing you can do to feel better or fix this situation."
- "You would be better off dead."
- "Other people would be better off if you were dead."
- "If you die by suicide, your friends and family will get over it."

All of the above thoughts are *factually untrue.*

While suicidal thinking is different for different people, a common element for many people is that the thoughts hit them like a wave. The thoughts start at a low level, gradually build to a peak, and then eventually start to diminish. This could occur over a matter of seconds, minutes, or hours.

4. Lewis, *Collected Letters*, 606.
5. Burns, *Feeling Good*, 385–86.

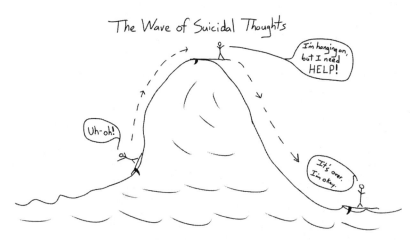

**The person on the surfboard is riding an intense wave of suicidal thoughts.
Effective safety plans get implemented at the "Uh oh!" part of the wave.**

Often amid thoughts of suicide, a person thinks of death as a logical solution. That is because people develop a sort of tunnel vision in their thinking. They forget about or dismiss the consequences of their actions. They forget about their future goals. They don't factor in the negative impact on their family or friends. When that wave of suicidal thoughts later decreases and their thinking expands, they often say to themselves, "What was I thinking? I wouldn't do that to my family or my friends! I have goals for my future."

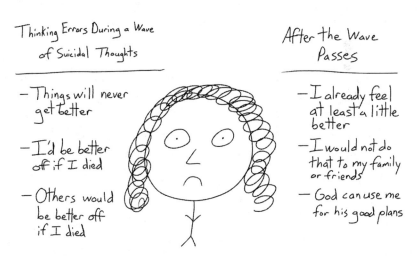

Safety Plans Save Lives

Safety plans are not perfect, and they are not the only solution for people at risk for suicide, but they are an essential tool. The best safety plans allow people to take action, to follow a sequence of steps (positive activities) that are under their control to stay safe until the wave of suicidal thoughts goes down. It is critical to start the positive steps at the beginning of the wave of suicidal thoughts. Once you reach the peak of the wave, it is very difficult to start the positive steps.

The best safety planning form that I have found to prevent suicide is the one used in the Safety Planning Intervention,[6] which was developed by Barbara Stanley, PhD, and Gregory Brown, PhD. I have included a Safety Plan form in the "Resources" section for you.

The steps of a good safety plan are as follows:

1. *Recognize Early Warning Signs*: This step is really about recognizing common triggers for thoughts of suicide. When the trigger hits, you should go to the next step and start working through your safety plan.

2. *Use Internal Coping Strategies*: Whatever you are doing, do something different. If that is not working, try another activity on your list for three to five minutes. Get up and shift your activities, repeatedly if necessary, to distract yourself from your negative thoughts. If this step is ineffective, move to the next step. If necessary, jump to step 5.

3. *Socialize for Support and to Reduce Isolation*: This step is the "don't be alone" step. Call or text someone and open a conversation. You could say something like, "Hey. What are you up to today? What do you have going on?" If this step is ineffective, move to the next step. If necessary, jump to step 5.

4. *Actively Seek Help from Family and Friends*: This is the step where you ask the go-to people in your life for help. You move from "Hey. What are you up to today?" to "I'm not doing well. I don't feel safe. I need some help." If this step is ineffective, move to the next step.

5. *Actively Seek Help from a Professional*: This is the step where you call your therapist, call your doctor, call or text 988 (the National Suicide Prevention Lifeline), dial 911, or go to the ER.

---

6. Stanley and Brown, "Safety Planning Intervention," 262.

6. *Reduce Access to Lethal Means*: It is completely logical to distance yourself from lethal means, such as firearms or a stash of pills, if you are at risk of suicide. The research is clear that firearm ownership increases the risk of suicide by firearm.[7] Let family and friends show that they care about you by safely storing your firearms temporarily when you are at a point in life when you are struggling with your safety.

There are many other safety plans, including ones available as smartphone apps. A very important step of any safety plan is to review it and improve it. If it looks like your safety plan is inadequate, see it as an opportunity to go over it again and improve it, because for many people safety plans do work and are very helpful.

Suicide Is an Irreversible, Devastating Choice for Temporary Problems

Depression is treatable. Did you catch that? Depression, the major cause of suicide, is *treatable*. Also, suicidal thoughts are temporary. There is a logical conclusion to be found here. Dying by suicide is a poor choice. Suicide is an extreme reaction to a temporary, fixable problem.

If you disagree with me on these points, consider some of the other reasons suicide is a poor choice. Suicide attempts can and do fail. What happens if you are permanently disabled because your suicide attempt did not work out as planned? This happens! Traumatic injury and survival are possibilities. There is also the possibility that a person who attempts suicide will change their mind after it is too late to turn back.

If you have depression or any other mental illness that is contributing to thoughts of suicide, get professional help immediately. There are many effective treatments for depression that I will elaborate on in chapters 6, 7, and 8. Suicide is an overreaction to a temporary, solvable problem.

Taking Suicide off the Table

I've heard some people say that thoughts of suicide are comforting for them. It alleviates their overwhelming anxiety or angst. However, for most people, it is easily argued that recurrent thoughts of suicide are unhealthy.

7. Florentine and Crane, "Suicide Prevention," 1628–29.

Habitual suicidal thinking can poison a person's problem-solving abilities. The thought of suicide becomes the solution for everything—every bad experience, every relationship conflict, every negative emotion, every moment of self-hatred, and every pet peeve.

I try to get the people I work with to see recurrent thoughts of suicide as a bad habit that can become their routine fallback. If they can see this kind of thinking as a bad habit, they can work on gradually kicking it.

When suicidal thoughts do not resolve, it can be helpful for a person to meet with a therapist trained in dialectical behavior therapy (DBT). DBT is very effective at reducing the risk of suicide. Other forms of psychotherapy can also help reduce the risk of suicide.

Another strategy for addressing recurrent thoughts of suicide is to make an active decision not to end your life—ever. I have seen many people have a positive transformation in their depression treatment when they take the option of suicide off the table. People who tell themselves, "Suicide is not an option for me; that option is off the table," often see a dramatic improvement in their depression and safety, as it forces them to take the necessary steps to get better and find healthier solutions to their problems.

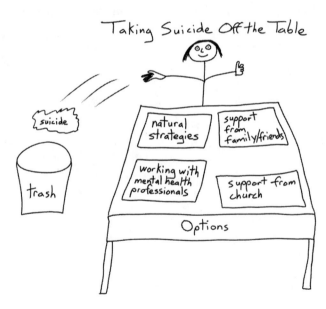

Taking Suicide Off the Table

suicide

trash

natural strategies

support from family/friends

working with mental health professionals

support from church

Options

Depression and Suicidal Thoughts Are Temporary, Solvable Problems

I want to encourage you to persevere. You are not a burden to others. You are unique and irreplaceable, and there is real hope and help for depression and suicidal thoughts. Consider that God is opposed to suicide and that suicide harms others. There are steps that you can take, like creating a safety plan, that allow you to actually do something about suicidal thoughts. If you struggle with thoughts of suicide, I would also encourage you to *decide to take the option of suicide off the table*, and watch how your thinking changes and treatment starts to become more effective. The following chapters in the next section will describe treatments that work, further providing proof that depression is treatable and getting free from depression is achievable.

Reflection

- Read 2 Corinthians 12:9–10. Do you believe this verse provides any guidance to Christians regarding the topic of suicide?

- Do you believe that God opposes suicide? Why or why not?

- Do you believe that suicide is self-murder? Why or why not?

- What do you think of the claim of depression expert Dr. David Burns that suicidal thinking is the result of a thinking error?

- What do you think about the list of the lies of depression that many suicidal people believe?

- Are there any steps that you plan to take as a result of reading this chapter (for example, sharing some of these ideas with others or completing a safety plan)?

II

Solutions
Dealing with Depression as a Christian

5

Building Your Team of Support

Each of you should use whatever gift you have received to serve others, as faithful stewards of God's grace in its various forms. (1 Peter 4:10)

Don't Go It Alone

EVEN IF YOU ARE smart and independent, you should not go through depression alone. There is a good chance that a specialist knows more than you about depression. Even doctors are encouraged not to provide their own medical care, as they could misinterpret or miss something due to being too close to the problem. You might think, "But I know myself the best." I can accept that perspective, but even if you know yourself better than anybody else in the world, that doesn't mean that you are also objective about yourself, especially when you are sick.

Consider these questions:

- If you were going in front of a judge, would you want a lawyer?
- If you had cancer, would you meet with a cancer specialist?

Dealing with the problems of depression alone puts you at risk, and working with a therapist or psychiatrist will likely dramatically improve your outcome. Relying only on yourself could result in your missing something important in the treatment of your mood or not being account-able. Getting to full freedom from depression (known as remission) is the goal of treatment because full remission allows you to thrive and reduces the chance you'll relapse.

If you develop depression, you need to hit it hard, get free of it, and keep it gone. If your depression only gets partly better, your prognosis is worse, as having leftover (residual) symptoms of depression predicts re-lapse and chronic depression.[1] You do not want chronic depression. A skilled team can help you get fully free from depression faster than you can on your own.

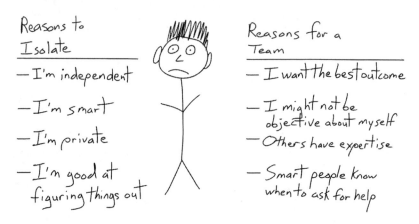

Reasons to
Isolate
— I'm independent
— I'm smart
— I'm private
— I'm good at
figuring things out

Reasons for a
Team
— I want the best outcome
— I might not be
objective about myself
— Others have expertise
— Smart people know
when to ask for help

There Are Effective and Ineffective Clinicians

There is a difference in quality among psychiatrists just as there is a differ-ence in quality among surgeons. There also is variability in the quality of psychotherapists. I'll talk more below about how to find skilled therapists and psychiatrists.

If you have depression, you need to find someone with both good *diagnostic* and *treatment* skills. Remember the equation from chapter 1: *wrong diagnosis = wrong treatment.*

For example, when my relative Sarah was hospitalized for severe de-pression, I called and left a message for Sarah's inpatient psychiatrist in the hopes that the team would take the time to carefully screen for hypomania (found in bipolar II disorder) and mania (found in bipolar I disorder). Un-fortunately, the doctor did not call me back and instead had a trainee call

1. Möller, "Outcomes," 102–05.

me. The trainee sounded bored and condescending, but I tried to make my point about the importance of getting Sarah's diagnosis correct to get her the best treatment. In a flat voice, the trainee said, "We already checked for all that." I shared with the trainee that I had already spoken to Sarah and, in fact, they had not screened her thoroughly. I figured that the trainee didn't have the necessary level of supervision, so I took the time to explain how to do the screening thoroughly and effectively. The trainee agreed to do the screening and report back. When she called back, her response was again abrupt. "We checked again, Dr. Lantz," she said, "It's not there," and then hung up. It turned out that she was wrong.

After a year of ineffective treatment of her depression, Sarah finally got the right diagnosis (bipolar II disorder) and the right treatment, after seeing more skilled clinicians.

The quality of care in psychiatry and the rest of mental health often boils down to education, training, and attitude. Unfortunately, some professionals do not strive for clinical excellence. They settle for being mediocre rather than being thorough. Another challenge in clinical care is when the mental health professionals only care about the immediate problem, not about long-term outcomes. Sarah's inpatient team appeared to only be concerned about depression and suicidal thoughts, so they mainly cared about getting her "undepressed" and discharged from the hospital. They did not seem to care about an accurate diagnosis or how their antidepressants would lead to mood instability a week or two after she was discharged from the hospital.

You can find clinicians who care about quality and who understand the importance of diagnosis. However, you also need to be alert for clinicians who do not seem to be thorough or who are satisfied with short-term, mediocre outcomes.

Team Members Can Enhance the Success of Treatment

You want your therapist and psychiatrist to be thorough and competent. In addition, you are likely to stick with treatment even when things get difficult if you have team members with the following traits:

Positive and encouraging: People with depression need to borrow hope from others until their hope comes back on its own. They need team members who are confident, who do not get demoralized, and who do not berate depressed people when they are struggling.

Active, not passive: Active team members will reach out to you if you are canceling meetings on them. It also is helpful to have team members who will schedule a time to meet with you rather than always leave it up to you to call them. If the routine response you get from a team member is, "Call me if you need me," and there is no scheduled time to connect, that team member is unlikely to be of much help.

Both natural and professional supports: A team does not need to be composed entirely of licensed professionals with degrees. A friend, relative, neighbor, coworker, boss, or pastor could all offer support to someone struggling with depression. For kids with severe depression, an approach called wraparound seeks to add more natural supports than professional supports on a team. If you are considering adding in more natural supports to get rid of severe depression but cannot think of who could help you, try answering the following questions:

- Who in your life is praying for you and checking in with you?

- Who in your life is willing to reach out to you if you start isolating yourself from others?

- Who is going to know if you are not taking care of your hygiene or other tasks, like paying your bills, going to work, or going to school?

Someone you know personally vs. someone new: I know several people with depression who simply have a hard time trusting someone with the personal details of their care unless they have already developed a personal relationship with the individual. Personally, I prefer not to blur the boundaries by becoming the doctor for my friends. It is easier for me to be objective in treatment if I am not also friends with my patients. Also, I enjoy separating myself from work when I'm trying to relax with my family and friends in the evening or on weekends. While it can be hard to confide in someone new, trust develops over time, and it's worth it to get free of depression.

Christians vs. people with other beliefs: I've had some patients whose first question is about my Christian faith. It has surprised me how important the answer to this question is for some people. I have seen such variability of quality of care among Christian and non-Christian psychiatrists and therapists alike that my approach has always been to determine first if a professional is simply any good at their job. If I was seeking mental health care for myself, that would be my first concern. If a non-Christian team member is asking challenging questions about your faith or values, then it would make sense for you to take the time to figure out if they are acting dismissively, criticizing your faith, or just trying to understand you better.

Empathy: Your team members must show empathy. How much are your team members attempting to see the world through your eyes? Now, that doesn't mean that they will agree with your perspective and do everything you want, but having team members who can understand your point of view is validating and enhances your connection with them.

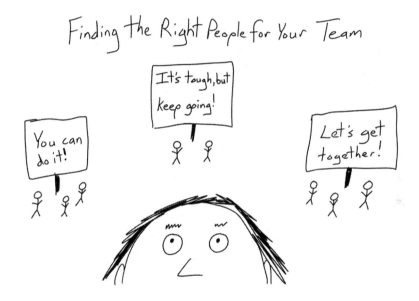

How to Find Quality Psychotherapy

The best strategy for finding a therapist is to talk to your primary care physician or your psychiatrist. It's very difficult to determine online who would be an excellent therapist, but one helpful measure is whether the therapist lists research-proven, evidence-based psychotherapeutic approaches that they consistently follow. I often encourage people to try out a new therapist by seeing them for at least three sessions. At the end of the third visit I have them ask themselves two questions:

"Do I feel like this therapist understands me and listens to me?"

"Is this therapist helping me / Do I believe that they can help me?"

If the answer to both questions is yes, you are likely to make progress in therapy. If the answer to either one of those questions is no, you are unlikely to make progress with this therapist, and it will likely be a waste of your time and money.

Keep in mind that your therapist should have you working on something in your life or practicing a skill between therapy visits. If your therapist is not having you do this, you may want to talk with your therapist about this or consider moving on to someone new. It is also helpful when working with a new therapist to talk about your treatment goals and ask them what type of treatment plan they would develop for you, what progress they would be looking for to determine when to end therapy, and an estimated timeline for the duration of therapy.

There is such a thing as low-quality therapy. "Crisis-of-the-week" (COW) therapy is a label often applied to low-quality talk therapy. This type of therapy tends to be reactive and to have no clear goals. No skills are taught or practiced. There may be excessive self-disclosure by the therapist.

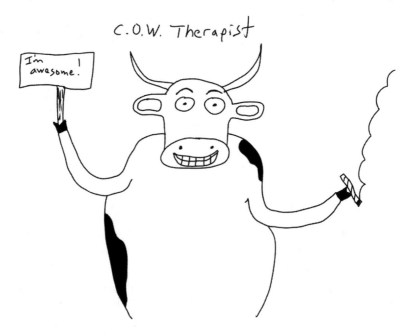

It's usually best to switch from a COW therapist to one with a deeper skill set.

COW therapy tends to be "tell me about your week," which is then discussed throughout the session, and near the end there is an insight or teachable moment imparted by the therapist to the client. This type of therapy often makes patients increasingly anxious, as they feel they have to keep the conversation going even when their life is going relatively well, so therapy may feel like a burden that the patient has to carry. They start to cancel and avoid therapy for reasons such as, "I don't have anything else to talk about. I don't know what else to say." If you find yourself involved in low-quality therapy, it is best to move on to a more qualified therapist.

How to Find a Good Psychiatrist

The internet will not tell you who the good psychiatrists are. This is because credentials, consumer rating sites, and resumes do not reliably indicate quality. The spectrum of quality within psychiatric care is substantial. High-quality psychiatric care is a combination of knowledge, competence, and interpersonal skills.

All is not lost in finding a good psychiatrist. Word of mouth in your community can be a very effective means of finding the best psychiatrist near you. The next best method is to schedule an appointment with one or more primary care physicians and ask them point-blank, "Who are the best psychiatrists in our community?" If the primary care physician looks uncomfortable or defensive and starts to name only psychiatrists who are in their hospital system, they are giving you bad information. If they smile and seem relaxed and can easily list the top one, two, or three psychiatrists in your community, you are in luck!

There is a shortage of psychiatrists in America, so your positive attitude, persistence, and flexibility in scheduling and payment will improve your chances of getting in to see someone good. If your preferred psychiatrist does not have immediate openings, you will need to get on their waitlist. Waitlists never get shorter unless you are on them. If the psychiatrist you want is closed to new patients, just leave them a friendly monthly voicemail to let them know you still desire an appointment.

Also, there is a growing workforce of psychiatric providers in the US, which mainly includes psychiatric nurse practitioners. Many psychiatric nurse practitioners are quite skilled and competent. However, as a medical doctor, a psychiatrist's medical training and experience are more extensive.

It's worth noting that primary care physicians prescribe the majority of antidepressants in the US, but their skill level and comfort level in treating depression may be limited. Some primary care physicians work in consultation with a psychiatrist in a model called collaborative care, which has excellent outcomes.

Getting Help to Get Better Faster

You can see tremendous progress in the treatment of depression if you have the right team. There are several factors to consider when building your team. Competence, empathy, proactiveness, and a positive attitude are just a few traits to look for in team members. Also, having a team member who is highly skilled in diagnosis is an absolute necessity. Using the strategies I have described can facilitate building your team and help you get fully free of depression.

Reflection

- Read 1 Peter 4:7–11, focusing especially on verse 10. Read Galatians 6:2. What do these verses say about trying to do everything yourself?
- If you were setting up a dream team of natural and professional supports for someone who had depression, how would you set it up? What people would you include?
- If you were looking for a mental health professional, would you start by looking at those with the best reputation and then hoping to find a Christian among them, or would you approach it the other way around? Why?
- Would you be willing to share the importance of your faith with a doctor/therapist who isn't a Christian?
- Do you think it would be easy or hard to find the kind of doctor or therapist you are looking for in your town? If you couldn't find the right person locally, would you be open to meeting someone by video, or is in-person treatment necessary? Why?
- Are there any steps that you plan to take as a result of reading this chapter (for example, lining up help for yourself, offering to help others, or looking into the availability of doctors or therapists in your community)?

6

Effective Natural Remedies
for Milder Depression

*You will go out in joy and be led forth in peace; the mountains
and hills will burst into song before you, and all the trees
of the field will clap their hands. (Isaiah 55:12)*

Moving Out of Your Comfort Zone

YOU WILL GET THE most out of this chapter by having an open attitude
about each solution presented. You might decide that some solutions are
not for you. Some of these strategies might take you out of your comfort
zone. At the end of this chapter, I hope that you will have found many positive surprises.

I'm going to be covering light therapy, yoga (including whole-body
heating), exercise, and behavioral activation strategies. I can tell you that
I've seen each of these interventions provide substantial improvement in
my patients' depression, and some have even reached freedom from depression by *only* using these strategies (as opposed to using more traditional treatments, which I cover in chapters 7, 8 and 9).

Quick disclaimer: *If you have suicidal thoughts or severe depression, then
you need to work with a professional and not rely on natural remedies alone.*

I have observed all four of the following interventions to be effective in clinical practice and medical research also shows these treatments to be helpful. The first two strategies, light therapy and yoga, have some medical research evidence showing their positive effects. The last two strategies, exercise and behavioral activation, have substantial evidence showing their positive impact on depression.

Light Therapy

Light therapy, or bright light therapy, is a treatment originally used to target seasonal affective disorder (SAD), a depressive disorder that tends to start in the fall, worsen in the winter, and lift in the spring. Most people know if they have SAD because they can feel the dread of it coming on as the days get shorter and the weather gets cooler in the fall.

In addition to sadness, people who experience SAD often have "atypical symptoms" of depression, such as extreme fatigue, increased appetite, and carbohydrate craving. The idea behind using light therapy to treat SAD is that it makes up for the lack of sunlight during the day, as the decreased light to our eyes is suspected to be the main cause of SAD. Bright light therapy is thought to have a corrective impact on the circadian rhythm and systems involving serotonin, melatonin, and CLOCK genes. Using bright light at the beginning of the day and correctly following other steps can be effective for many people who suffer from this form of depression.

For example, in one study, light therapy for SAD was as effective as an antidepressant.[1] In a more recent, large, placebo-controlled study of SAD,[2] it was found that both Prozac (fluoxetine) and light therapy were better than placebo in treating SAD and that the light therapy resulted in faster recovery and fewer side effects than Prozac.

My colleagues and I have seen in our own patients that some people experience a clear benefit from light therapy for their fall/winter depression while others do not. Unfortunately, the majority of people who attempt light therapy miss one or more critical steps. Maybe they bought the wrong light. Possibly the instructions were poor. More often than not, the reason that light therapy does not work is that the person using it does not sit close enough to the light, regularly enough, and for long enough. If you plan to attempt using light therapy, make sure to read my article "Light Therapy for

1. Ruhrmann et al., "Effects of Fluoxetine versus Bright Light," 926–29.
2. Lam et al., "The Can-SAD Study" 809–10.

Depression: Are You Doing It Right?" at my website (lenlantz.com/unJoy) to ensure that you are following the right steps.

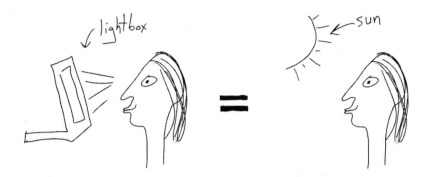

Keep in mind that if you have severe depression, light therapy alone is unlikely to be enough to help you. If you have a major mood disorder, it is a good idea to utilize light therapy under the supervision of a psychiatrist. If you have seasonal depression and it's winter, you owe it to yourself to determine if light therapy is effective for you.

Yoga

Get out of your comfort zone! I know that yoga can be a controversial topic for Christians, but don't write it off. During the meditation and mindfulness components of yoga classes, just pray silently. Be a shining light to those around you in yoga.

Medical research shows that yoga helps depression, and its benefits appear to range from mild to moderate. A recent meta-analysis of thirteen studies showed that yoga has a moderate effect on reducing depression and that shorter, more frequent sessions per week, as opposed to longer, less-frequent sessions, show greater benefit.[3] Yoga has also been shown to help depression in kids.[4]

Yoga classes have the additional benefit of stretching and strengthening your body (I am incredibly inflexible, so yoga is especially good for me). Some yoga classes are heated (hot yoga) and others are not. If you are a beginner, just remember to bring a mat, towel, water, and try not to grunt or moan too loudly (if you are vocally protesting, then you are probably

3. Brinsley et al., "Effects of Yoga," 994–98.

4. James-Palmer et al., "Yoga as an Intervention," 3–12.

overdoing the exercises). If you have anxiety about going, you can go with a friend. For example, I convinced my Christian buddy Kevin to join me one day. For some reason, he absolutely refused to call it "yoga" afterward and would only refer to it as "limbering."

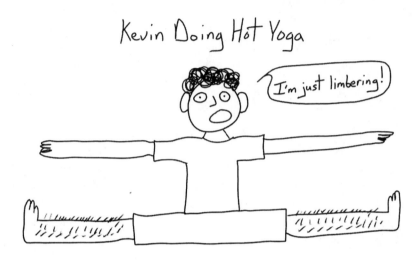

Yoga is very much about slowing down and taking care of yourself. When you engage in self-care, a cascade of other positive things happens. Yoga can be calm and restorative or very physically demanding. Many people express feelings of improved emotional and physical well-being after completing a yoga practice. There is a significant amount of inertia—physical and mental—that occurs in depression. Yoga combats this inertia through physical movement and mental activation. Yoga is very much a mind-body activity. It takes determination to hold poses in yoga because sometimes it's uncomfortable. Working through the discomfort takes concentration and perseverance.

I especially enjoy doing hot yoga because I believe the heat is beneficial. For decades, researchers have been looking at whole-body heating (through the use of hot baths or infrared heating) for the treatment of depression. A recent study used infrared whole-body heating over six weeks for people with depression.[5] People who received active treatment did better than the placebo, and the group collectively experienced around a 50 percent reduction in depressive symptoms. Researchers concluded it was

5. Janssen et al., "Whole-Body Hyperthermia," 792–94.

a "safe and rapidly acting modality," although more evidence is needed for this to be accepted as the standard of care in the field of psychiatry.

Some people are cautious about yoga as they do not feel comfortable with the meditative parts of the class. Most yoga studios in America are not religious but are instead communities that behave like an extended network of friends. Who are the people who attend yoga regularly? I can only speak to the studio I go to, where sometimes I'm the only guy in the class. The studio I go to has a handful of guys who regularly attend but is mostly filled with women, many of whom are professional leaders in my town. And if meditation is part of a class you attend, you can choose to focus on whatever you like, such as a prayer or a Bible verse.

I remember the first time I went to a hot yoga studio. I thought to myself, "Are they going to try to make me chant? Because I am *not* going to chant! And I'm not going to take my shirt off even if the instructor tells me to." My unfounded concerns about going to yoga never came to pass. I worried that I was too inflexible or that I would be judged. The thing about yoga is that you are supposed to be paying attention to yourself, not others. What others are doing should not matter to you in the least. Therefore, you have the opportunity to be happy with any progress you make because you are not comparing your body, abilities, or progress to anyone else, including the teacher. They call it yoga *practice*, not performance.

Exercise

The research on exercise for depression is consistently positive. But you will need to accept that you cannot wait for energy or motivation to show up so that you feel like exercising. Reality requires that you first start moving your body and then energy and motivation will naturally increase later.

When you are depressed, you often feel stuck. People with depression frequently don't exercise because their energy and motivation are so low. Just brushing your teeth can feel like a major chore when you are depressed. However, there is hope. Most people do not understand how much they can benefit from a small amount of exercise.

It can be incredibly easy to enjoy the physical and mental health benefits of exercise. Federal guidelines for exercise show how straightforward exercise can be. Walking, dancing, playing, and running all count. Moderate-intensity exercise means anything that gets your heart beating faster, and muscle-strengthening activity just means that you are making your muscles work harder than usual. That's it! Exercise need not be demanding. It does not require a tennis racket, mountain bike, or gym membership.

While there are dozens of research studies showing that exercise exerts a positive effect on major depression, the medical community has been slow to embrace exercise as a treatment for depression. In 1999, the research study "Effects of Exercise Training on Older Patients with Major Depression" was published.[6] The results showed that sixteen weeks of exercise produced similar benefits to the antidepressant Zoloft (sertraline) for people with major depression ranging from mild to severe intensity. The people in the exercise arm of the study just needed to walk or jog three times per week for forty-five minutes for sixteen weeks. There was another major finding. If patients from the 1999 study continued to exercise for another six months, they were half as likely to relapse back into depression compared to those who stopped exercising.[7] In other words, the benefits of exercise stop when you stop exercising.

So, exercise was shown to help depression and the entire field of medicine erupted in celebration, right? Wrong.

These incredible researchers were met with skepticism and denial. The larger medical community could not believe the enormity of their results. They raised objections about how accurate the diagnoses of depression were, how the study was not blinded, and that there was no placebo control in the study.

So, many of the same researchers from the 1999 study put together a more rigorous research protocol called the SMILE study.[8] In this study, the researchers compared the exercise group to Zoloft and placebo (sugar pill) groups. The researchers found that the "unadjusted remission rates were: supervised exercise = 45%; home-based exercise = 40%; medication = 47%; and placebo = 31%."[9]

The effect of exercise was similar to that of Zoloft. Both exercise and Zoloft beat the placebo. Exercise clearly helps major depression! Also, a one-year continuation study showed that continuing the treatment for another year resulted in 67 percent remission in the exercise groups and

6. Blumenthal et al., "Effects of Exercise," 2351–53.
7. Babyak et al., "Exercise Treatment," 634–36.
8. Blumenthal et al., "Exercise and Pharmacotherapy," 591–94.
9 Blumenthal et al., "Exercise and Pharmacotherapy," 592.

63 percent remission in the Zoloft group.[10] In other words, the longer you exercise, the greater the benefit for depression.

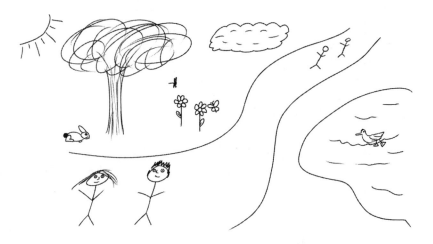

Exercise for depression literally can be as easy as a brisk walk in the park.

Behavioral Activation

Behavioral activation is the process of proactively increasing your positive activity level. This strategy for depression is consistent with the Christian faith. Being busy all day doing positive activities that align with your values can help your depression immensely.

In a meta-analysis research study in 2009, behavioral activation was shown to be substantially beneficial compared to placebo in the treatment of depression.[11] Behavioral activation can help major depression tremendously and can also be a strategy to prevent mental illness in times of stress and uncertainty, such as the loss of a job, having a child, the loss of a loved one, or other major life transitions or disruptions, including quarantine during a pandemic.

I have heard countless stories from friends, family, and patients about the negative impact on their mood after transitioning from a high activity level to a low activity level. Think about the times in your life when your

10. Hoffman et al, "One-Year Follow-Up of the SMILE," 128–31.
11. Mazzucchelli et al., "Behavioral Activation," 399–404.

mood crashed after a major accomplishment or task. Shouldn't you have been on cloud nine? The drop in mood could be related to your life being completely out of balance and your feeling exhausted by the time you completed your goal or project, but it also could be due to moving from a high activity level to a low activity level or moving from a structured, goal-oriented schedule to no schedule at all. You can protect your mental health during these times through behavioral activation.

When someone is depressed, they lack energy, motivation, and enjoyment, which leads them to stop doing the activities that normally help them feel good. Their resulting inactivity then worsens their depression. When adding activities to your schedule, try to broaden your range of activities, maybe including things that are opposite ends of the spectrum or that engage all of your senses (sight, smell, touch, taste, hearing):

- Social and solitude.
- Nature and indoors.
- Art and puzzles.
- Playing music and listening to music.
- Physical activity and prayer.
- Entertainment activities and meaningful service.

A sample of activities that can be used in behavioral activation include:

- Go for a walk in nature and spend some of that time in prayer.
- Call a friend.
- Attend a Bible study.
- Draw a picture or doodle.
- Play your favorite song and sing along with it (no matter how good or bad you are at singing).
- Join a morning social coffee group.
- Go to a museum.
- Visit a flower shop or a greenhouse.
- Plan to visit a new restaurant or get takeout.
- Complete a puzzle, sudoku, or crossword puzzle.

Behavioral activation is about forcing yourself to do meaningful activities that are in line with your values—the things you do when you're not depressed. When a depressed person puts themselves on a schedule filled with positive activities, they send powerful signals to their brain to wake up and function. A busy schedule with cognitive activation makes the brain function in a non-depressed way and stimulates neural pathways that are underactive in depression. And even if someone with depression doesn't experience as much enjoyment as normal with positive activities, chances are they will feel better than they would have if they had done nothing.

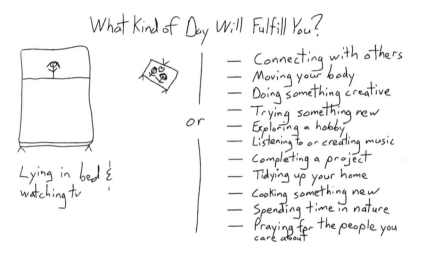

What Kind of Day Will Fulfill You?

Lying in bed & watching tv

or

— Connecting with others
— Moving your body
— Doing something creative
— Trying something new
— Exploring a hobby
— Listening to or creating music
— Completing a project
— Tidying up your home
— Cooking something new
— Spending time in nature
— Praying for the people you care about

Start Natural Treatments for Depression Today

The first step of using natural strategies for depression is simply to begin. Start a natural strategy today and choose not to judge yourself on your effort or perceived success. If you do anything at all, I am happy to tell you that you have succeeded. The challenge is that you will need to continue these strategies every day for them to be effective. Doing anything when you are depressed can seem like a monumental task, especially if your energy and motivation are very low. However, starting the activity itself will develop your internal motivation and energy over time. So, start light therapy if you are in the fall/winter season and you believe it is right for you. Consider yoga and get out of your comfort zone. If you are physically inactive, start by walking—that's all you have to do, then everything will follow naturally from there. Behavioral activation is incredibly powerful for depression.

Put together today's schedule with activities that are the most in alignment with your values. When facing depression, the process of getting better can seem overwhelming or leave a person feeling out of control. The natural strategies above are all about doing effective behaviors that are under your control to improve your mood.

Reflection

- Read Isaiah 55:12. What does this verse make you think about? Consider the interplay of nature and emotions in this verse.

- Do you think that using light therapy could help someone who is only depressed in the fall and winter seasons? Why or why not?

- What is your reaction to the information on yoga? Could you see yourself doing yoga and benefitting from it?

- What comes to your mind when you imagine yourself exercising? Are there any types of exercise that you especially enjoy?

- Were you surprised to learn about the power of behavioral activation exercises? If you had a free day in your town and were instructed to fill your day any way you chose, as long as those activities were in alignment with your values, what five or ten things would you do that day?

- Are there any steps that you plan to take as a result of reading this chapter (for example, starting exercising by walking, talking a friend into exercising with you, creating a list of behavioral activation strategies, or reading an article found at lenlantz.com/unJoy)?

7

Therapy Can Really Help Depression

Two are better than one, because they have a good return for their labor: If either of them falls down, one can help the other up. But pity anyone who falls and has no one to help them up. (Ecclesiastes 4:9–10)

Therapy for Depression

THERAPY IS ONE OF the most effective treatments for depression and anxiety. While you can address many goals in therapy, one of the purposes is to share and unburden yourself of pent-up thoughts and feelings. Another reason to do therapy is to convince yourself that life is more bearable and to learn some coping skills. Most importantly, therapy can help you gain a greater understanding of the thoughts that drive feelings of misery and hopelessness.

There are many different forms of psychotherapy, more than I can cover in this chapter. While there are many useful forms of psychotherapy and it is certainly the case that different styles of psychotherapy are a good fit for different people, the ultimate benefit of any form of psychotherapy can be distilled down to the skill and responsiveness of the therapist. Whether or not psychotherapy—any style of psychotherapy—is effective for any person boils down to two critical factors:[1]

- The *therapeutic alliance*: Many studies have shown that the strength of the therapeutic alliance (the connection/fit between patient and therapist) is one of the best predictors of success in therapy.[2]

- Frequent feedback on *therapeutic outcomes*: Psychotherapy is more effective when the patient can honestly share with the therapist the amount of progress they are experiencing.[3]

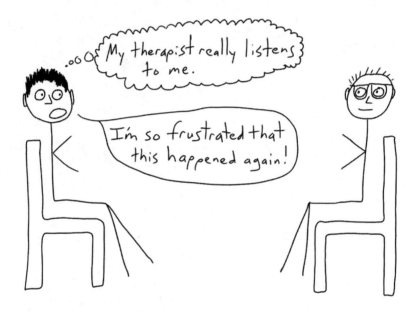

The best outcomes in therapy result from empathy expressed by the therapist, the strength of the therapeutic relationship, and feedback from the depressed person to the therapist regarding their progress. Separate from the time commitment and financial considerations of doing therapy, there is another cost to doing therapy, which is taking a risk by sharing what is going on in your life with another person. It's not always easy to do therapy.

1. Miller et al. "Outcome of Psychotherapy," 91–93.

2. Horvath and Symonds, "Working Alliance," 141–46; Krupnick et al., "Therapeutic Alliance," 535–36.

3. Lambert et al., "Therapists with Feedback," 57–62; Reese et al., "Continuous Feedback System," 423–27.

For example, I recall one of my teen patients calling me and telling me that she decided to start therapy, to which I replied, "Good job!" She had avoided therapy for years and was literally moaning as she told me that she would now take my advice but was not looking forward to it. She, like many of my other patients, was later pleasantly surprised that therapy was helpful for her depression and she began to look forward to the therapy meetings.

Therapy Is Not Anti-Christian

Many Christian patients have expressed to me that they are anxious about working with a non-Christian therapist. As this is a dealbreaker for some people, I am happy to provide patients the names and phone numbers of excellent Christian therapists in my community. At the same time, I counsel my patients that high-caliber therapists can work with people who have a variety of values and beliefs that they may not share themselves. Consider for a second that not all Christians or Christian denominations share all the same beliefs. Skilled therapists are able to work with people from a variety of backgrounds and faiths and help each individual with their depression in a manner that honors the patient's values and worldview.

Psychotherapy, when appropriately performed by the therapist, is not against the Christian faith. I am unaware of any form of mainstream psychotherapy that has an objective to attack Christianity or convert Christians to humanism or atheism.

The Most Effective Forms of Therapy Usually Teach Skills

Cognitive behavioral therapy (CBT) is arguably one of the most effective forms of face-to-face psychotherapy. It is time-limited, focuses on skills-building, and works to rebalance thoughts. Most of the time that a person experiences an emotion, such as happiness or anxiety, a thought preceded and triggered the emotion. Chronic unwanted emotions that are out of proportion to situations are usually caused by recurring unbalanced thoughts. CBT works to rebalance or replace the unbalanced thoughts and results in a person having emotional responses that are more in tune with their life circumstances. This often leads to a substantial reduction in excessive sadness, anxiety, and anger. Here are some of the most thoroughly studied forms of psychotherapy for depression, including a less well-known variant of CBT designed for Christians, called religious cognitive behavioral therapy (RCBT):

Cognitive Behavioral Therapy (CBT): This form of therapy is similar to coaching because it is almost entirely focused on the present and on skills building. The types of skills that people learn in CBT include identifying the difference between thoughts and emotions, practicing coping skills, learning techniques to manage anxiety and other negative emotions, and cognitive reframing, which uses thought logs to replace automatic negative thoughts with balanced thoughts, which in turn balance emotions.

Religious (Christian) Cognitive Behavioral Therapy (RCBT): This form of therapy is a variant of CBT that directly incorporates the Bible and Christian values. RCBT involves the active use of religious beliefs as a foundation to identify and replace unbalanced thoughts to reduce depression. RCBT for Christians is thought to be at least as effective as traditional CBT at treating depression, and a 2016 study found that RCBT was especially effective among highly religious clients.[4]

Acceptance and Commitment Therapy (ACT): This form of therapy is about action and uses a combination of CBT and behavior therapy. ACT focuses on the use of acceptance and mindfulness strategies in combination with behavioral and commitment strategies to help people see positive movement in different areas of their life. ACT encourages you to state your values, assess where your life is at in relation to your values, and make commitments to yourself about what you plan to do about where you are in life. ACT is a thoroughly researched therapy and is likely one of the therapy modalities most supportive of Christians as it is highly values-focused.

Dialectical Behavior Therapy (DBT): This is a form of CBT that focuses on helping people with suicidal thoughts and self-defeating behaviors. DBT teaches a variety of skills and helps people to radically accept themselves just as they are while at the same time seeking positive change.

Interpersonal Therapy (IPT): This form of therapy is usually the most effective for people who are dealing with problems such as loss/grief, relationship problems, and role transitions. IPT can be very effective for the treatment of depression.

Supportive Psychotherapy: This form of therapy, which is often referred to as "treatment as usual" in research, is also effective when performed by a skilled therapist. While there is far less research available on supportive psychotherapy than many other therapies, it has been studied and found to

4. Koenig et al., "Religiously-Integrated," 237–53.

help symptoms of depression.[5] Supportive psychotherapy uses a variety of approaches, including encouraging the use of adaptive coping strategies, improving self-esteem, and creating a "safe space" or place to deal with difficult thoughts, emotions, and life experiences.

Non-Face-to-Face Options

Not every person who wants help is interested in or able to participate in face-to-face therapy. There are several potential barriers to face-to-face therapy (whether in person or by video) that can be more easily addressed with Internet-based cognitive behavioral therapy (iCBT). Different forms of iCBT use the same strategies as conventional CBT and may involve interaction with a trained therapist or be entirely automated. iCBT might involve many activities, such as watching videos, reading about helpful strategies, doing thought-balancing exercises, engaging in stress-reduction activities, and tracking progress.

Internet-based cognitive behavioral therapy (iCBT) can be more suitable for some people than traditional therapy. It can be a solution for people who want and could be helped by CBT but are not able to find it in their communities, can't attend therapy sessions during the hours therapists are available, or struggle to afford the cost of therapy. Also, iCBT is self-paced, so it can work with nearly any person's schedule. In a meta-analysis of thirteen studies of self-guided iCBT compared to controls, the iCBT treatment was found to be significantly more effective in treating depression.[6]

Forgiveness and Forgiveness Therapy

The final type of therapy I want to discuss involves depression that was triggered or maintained due to a conflict or disagreement with another person. If this is the case for you, you might feel very stuck about what to do, especially if you feel that you are unable to move forward until the other person apologizes or if you simply feel unable to forgive the other person. Even if the other person genuinely apologized, you might still find it hard to forgive them.

5. Cuijpers et al., "Supportive Therapy," 283–89.
6. Karyotaki et al., "Internet-Based," 353–56.

Be kind and compassionate to one another, forgiving each other, just as in Christ God forgave you. (Ephesians 4:32)

If there is one thing that I have suggested to patients that has most often offended them, even among Christians, it has been my suggestion that they consider the idea of forgiveness or forgiveness therapy. Past trauma can exert an incredibly powerful effect not just on mood but also on people's entire lives. Forgiving others might be one of the hardest commandments found in the Bible. Even when it appears appropriate and obvious, people can feel very threatened by the idea that forgiveness might be necessary to completely free them from their depression.

For if you forgive other people when they sin against you, your heavenly Father will also forgive you. But if you do not forgive others their sins, your Father will not forgive your sins. (Matthew 6:14–15)

It's clear what the Bible says about forgiveness. We should do it, but it can be hard to do. I believe that one of the best Christian books on forgiveness is *Total Forgiveness* by R. T. Kendall. I have personally found forgiving others to be incredibly powerful in my life, and it has allowed me to give up past grudges and no longer see people who harmed me as adversaries. However, knowing that we are to forgive each other and our enemies is easy to say and hard to do. For example, I have given *Total Forgiveness* to several relatives who are strong Christians who struggle with their mood due to relationship problems. The common response I get is, "It's too hard." It is clear to me that difficulty forgiving or the inability to forgive others is a barrier to improving depression.

I can do all this through him who gives me strength. (Philippians 4:13)

Studies of forgiveness therapy show that "forgiving a variety of real-life interpersonal offenses can be effective in promoting different dimensions of mental well-being."[7] Research demonstrates that forgiveness therapy results in improvements in depression, anger, hostility, stress, and distress. It also increases positive affect (such as satisfaction, happiness, gratitude, confidence, hopefulness, and energy).

---

7. Akhtar and Barlow, "Forgiveness Therapy," 107.

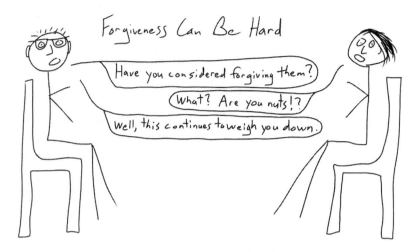

Therapy Helps Depression and Can Be Done in Alignment with Christian Beliefs

Therapy is one of the most effective treatments for depression. There are many forms of therapy and there can be substantial variability in the skill each therapist has in delivering the most effective forms of therapy. In the end, it comes down to a few elements that determine whether or not you will make progress in therapy. While some Christians insist on working only with a Christian therapist, others are comfortable working with a skilled therapist who will learn, respect, and encourage them to find and use strategies that are in alignment with their faith. Just as no two Christians are alike, the same is true for therapists. It takes courage to pursue therapy, trust another person, and take steps in your spiritual life, such as forgiving another person. It can be done. You can achieve full freedom from depression and learn skills for coping with negative thoughts and emotions.

Reflection

- Read Ecclesiastes 4:9–10. Do you believe the help described in the verses could apply to receiving counseling about emotions? Why or why not?
- Which types of therapy seem most appealing to you?
- Would you ever start psychotherapy if you felt you needed it?

- If you felt you needed therapy, would you be more likely to work with a person or with a computer program like iCBT? Why?

- What are your views on forgiveness and forgiveness therapy? Do you think you could ever forgive someone if they did not first apologize?

- Are there any steps that you plan to take as a result of reading this chapter (for example, reading a book on forgiveness or finding out if there are any good therapists in your community)?

8

The Ins and Outs of Medications for Depression

Plans fail for lack of counsel, but with many advisers they succeed. (Proverbs 15:22)

Do Antidepressants Help Depression?

ANTIDEPRESSANTS CAN SUBSTANTIALLY HELP mild, moderate, and severe forms of depression. Ask anyone you know who has taken an antidepressant for their depression, and if they are still on it, they just might tell you that they cannot function without it or that it saved their life.

Having said that, antidepressants are not a cure-all. They do not necessarily change your thoughts or cause behaviors that could also lead to the improvement of your depression. For example, antidepressants do not force you to:

- Exercise.

- Go to bed and get up at scheduled times.

- Learn how to balance your thoughts through psychotherapy.

- Eliminate repetitive, hours-long naps.

- Eat a healthy, balanced diet.

- Fill your schedule with meaningful activities.

- Reduce or eliminate substances that are unhealthy for you, such as nicotine, alcohol, or cannabis.

- Fix other problems in your life, such as chronic pain or other medical conditions.

Do you see where I'm going with this? Antidepressants can really help you, but medications alone might not fix depression.

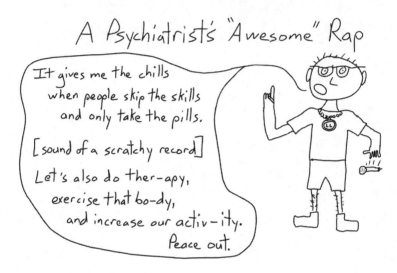

A Psychiatrist's "Awesome" Rap

It gives me the chills
when people skip the skills
and only take the pills.

[sound of a scratchy record]

Let's also do ther-apy,
exercise that bo-dy,
and increase our activ-ity.
Peace out.

Antidepressants have been proven in medical research to alleviate and eliminate depression in patients. Each prescription antidepressant has been approved by the US Food & Drug Administration (FDA) after multiple research studies show it to be safe and effective. Antidepressant medications are found to be more effective than a placebo (sugar pill) in the treatment of depression. However, there are a couple of challenges with medical research:

1. The placebo response rates in research studies have been high, so the benefit from antidepressants is often incrementally better but not enormously better than a placebo.

2. There have been very few good long-term studies comparing antidepressants to placebo. The studies that call into question whether or

not antidepressants work for depression are basing their results on short-term studies when the power of the placebo effect is at its peak.[1]

You might be asking yourself, "If antidepressants are only incrementally better than placebos, should I just take a placebo if I'm depressed?" My answer to you is that the best practices and current clinical guidelines still recommend antidepressants for depression. Future research will provide greater clarity as to whether placebo responses in studies have been artificially high and whether the placebo response drops off shortly after the initial benefit. More research needs to be done to better understand current antidepressants and find better antidepressants in the future.

Because I have a clinical focus and expertise in treating treatment-resistant depression, I am well aware of the limitations of antidepressant medications; however, I have seen that antidepressants can and do save lives. While antidepressants do not help everyone, they can exert tremendous benefit. Antidepressant medications can and do work for depression, and when they don't work or stop working, there are other, very effective options that will be discussed in chapter 9. Based on my medical education and clinical experience, if I had substantial depression, I would definitely try an antidepressant medication.

What Antidepressants Do to Your Mood

Some people joke around and call their antidepressant their "happy pill," but everyone who has been on an antidepressant knows that is not how it works. You don't take an antidepressant on Monday and feel happy that day, then skip the medication on Tuesday and feel sad.

Antidepressant medications gradually alleviate depression, but do not directly cause a person to feel happy. The benefit comes from taking the medication every day, resulting in gradual improvement over the course of weeks. Kids tend to have the fastest response. The elderly tend to have the slowest response to antidepressants, and other adults are somewhere in between.

The goal of treatment with an antidepressant is to allow you to get back to your normal, baseline mood. Some people worry that an antidepressant could change their personality. That certainly is not the goal, and a personality change would be considered an unwanted side effect. For

1. Hengartner et al., "Placebo-Controlled Trials," 5–8.

example, the father of one of my patients initially refused to have an antidepressant prescribed for his severely depressed teenage daughter because of his past experience with an antidepressant. He said, "Antidepressants don't work! They only make you numb and stop caring." When I was able to fully explain to him that what he experienced was a side effect, that his experience would not likely be replicated in his daughter, and that we would stop the medication if she had that kind of side effect, he changed his mind and we started antidepressant treatment (and she did great). The ultimate goal of treatment is to achieve full freedom from depression (remission) and to get that improvement to last.

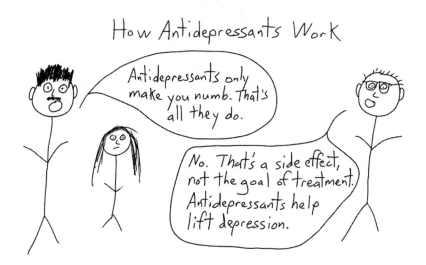

You can work with your doctor in medication selection depending on which symptoms are causing you the most trouble. For example, if you have anxiety, you might not start with Wellbutrin (bupropion), as the medication can increase anxiety in a substantial portion of people. Or, you might try to leverage the side effects of a medication to your advantage. In the case of depression and insomnia, you might consider Zoloft (sertraline) at bedtime, as the medication can be sedating, or Prozac (fluoxetine) in the morning, as the medication perks up some people during the day.

Types of Antidepressant Medications

I've been surprised over time to see how many depressed patients have never had full trials of more than one antidepressant medication. A full trial means taking a medication for a long enough time and increasing to the maximum dose if lower doses are not fully effective. Not all psychiatric medications treat depression, and mood-stabilizing medications can be of limited benefit in the treatment of major depression. While augmenting strategies, such as adding lithium, thyroid hormone, an anticonvulsant, or a new generation antipsychotic medicine to a person's current antidepressant medication, can help treatment-resistant depression, such medications are unlikely to be effective for major depression in the absence of an antidepressant.

There are different categories of antidepressants that differently affect levels of neurotransmitters in the brain, primarily serotonin, norepinephrine, and dopamine. While it can be helpful to take two antidepressant medications from different categories, it does not make sense to simultaneously take two antidepressants from the same category. Common categories and medications are:

- SSRI: Prozac (fluoxetine), Zoloft (sertraline), Celexa (citalopram), Lexapro (escitalopram), Paxil (paroxetine), Luvox (fluvoxamine).
- SNRI: Effexor (venlafaxine), Cymbalta (duloxetine), Pristiq (desvenlafaxine), Fetzima (levomilnacipran).
- NDRI: Wellbutrin (bupropion).
- Serotonin modulator: Remeron (mirtazapine), Viibryd (vilazodone), Trintellix (vortioxetine).
- Tricyclic: amitriptyline, nortriptyline, and others.
- MAOI: tranylcypromine and others.

There are fewer medications that specifically help bipolar depression. In general, it is recommended that you work with a specialist, such as a psychiatrist, if you have bipolar disorder. Most psychiatrists do not recommend an antidepressant alone for the treatment of bipolar depression, since this can lead to significant mood instability, hypomania/mania, or worsened depression overall.

Some of the medications that can be effective for bipolar depression include Lamictal (lamotrigine), lithium, Latuda (lurasidone), Seroquel (quetiapine), Vraylar (cariprazine), Caplyta (lumateperone), and Symbyax (a combination of olanzapine and fluoxetine).

General Approaches to Medication Changes

Many people don't know how often their antidepressants should be changed when they have not achieved remission. The best teachers I had in medical school and residency routinely reminded me of two basic rules to guide me in the treatment of my patients:

1. If it ain't broke, don't fix it (Interpretation: if your current treatment is working, don't change it).

2. If it's broke, fix it (Interpretation: if your current treatment isn't working, it's time for a change).

I realize that does not sound complicated; however, sometimes doctors violate these basic, common-sense rules. There is a third rule that I always try to follow as well, which is:

3. Only change one thing at a time.

If you changed two or more medications at the same time and experienced side effects, you might not know what caused the side effects. If you changed more than one medication and experienced symptom improvement, you might not know what caused the improvement. If your doctor routinely makes more than one medication change at a time, it might be time for you to find a new doctor (see chapter 5 for how to find a good psychiatrist).

The "Scientific" Approach to Med Changes

1. If it ain't broke, don't fix it.

2. If it's broke, fix it.

3. Only change 1 thing at a time.

Genetic Testing Can Be Helpful in the Treatment of Depression

Genetic testing is not currently advanced to the point of telling you what diagnosis you have or what medication will help your depression. However, it can provide useful clinical information. Genetic testing (or pharmacogenetic testing) primarily helps show how the liver breaks down psychiatric medication through different enzyme pathways. Most medications are broken down through two to five of these enzyme pathways. If one of these enzymes has an abnormality in the genes encoding it, the enzyme won't work as well. Therefore, the medication will not be broken down and removed from the body as quickly as predicted, and the blood level of the medication will rise to higher levels and possibly cause more side effects or even toxicity. At the other end of the spectrum, if there are extra copies of genes that encode these enzymes, the extra enzymes will break down medications very quickly, preventing a person from benefiting from the medication because they can't get the medication up to a therapeutic blood level.

If you have tried several antidepressant medications and you have seen no benefit or have experienced serious side effects, genetic testing may provide you with some answers and some guidance. It can help predict if you will have side effects or explain why previous medication trials weren't effective. Parents who are considering starting their child on a psychiatric medication may also pursue genetic testing. The testing will not necessarily tell them whether a specific medication will help their child or not, but it may help determine ahead of time which medications pose the greatest risk of side effects.

Newer Treatments for Depression

One of the newest medication treatments for depression is ketamine delivered intravenously (IV) or by a nasal spray. While ketamine primarily is used in higher doses for anesthesia, at lower doses IV ketamine can rapidly (though usually temporarily) improve depressive symptoms and resolve suicidal thoughts. Despite the research evidence showing that IV ketamine is effective in the treatment of depression, it does not yet have FDA approval for the treatment of depression.[2]

2. aan het Rot et al., "Intravenous Ketamine," 141–42.

Medical research has also shown that ketamine nasal spray, Spravato (esketamine), is effective when used in conjunction with an antidepressant, and it has received approval by the FDA for the treatment of depression.[3] A significant percentage of people have seen substantial benefits from both IV and nasal forms of ketamine. There are temporary, common side effects that are monitored with ketamine treatment, for example dissociation (feeling disconnected from your body) and elevations in blood pressure.

Other substances, such as the hallucinogen psilocybin, are being studied as possible treatments for depression, but more research is needed before such substances are approved for widespread clinical use in the treatment of depression.[4]

Sobriety Can Help Your Mood

People can struggle significantly with addictive substances that can affect mood, examples being cannabis (marijuana), alcohol, and other chemicals. And it can be hard for people to be objective about the true effects of these substances on their mood, anxiety, relationships, and functioning. In my work, I have gotten to know many people who struggle with addictions. Usually, people are not objective about their drug use until after they become sober.

Increased use of alcohol is associated with an increased risk of depression.[5] This makes sense, as alcohol is a central nervous system depressant. What might come as a surprise to you is that cannabis use disorder is associated with *triple the rates* of depression and anxiety.[6] I've brought up this research to my patients who are addicted to cannabis and most tell me that these results cannot be true. Many of them believe that cannabis is the only thing that has ever helped their mood. My best guess is that many of them are confusing the short-lived high of intoxication with long-term benefit. They are focused on short-term gain and missing the fact that they are declining over the long term. I have seen more than one patient with cannabis addiction become sober. Their mood improved with sobriety and they were able to see that sobriety was at least partially responsible for the improvement of their mood.

3. Daly et al., "Intranasal Esketamine," 141–44.
4. Davis et al., "Psilocybin-Assisted Therapy," 485–87.
5. Boden and Fergusson, "Alcohol and Depression," 907–11.
6. Onaemo et al., "Comorbid Cannabis Use," 469–71.

Chronic substance users may not see the negative effects of substances in their lives because their focus is on an immediate, temporary emotional change, not long-term outcomes and consequences. Consider substance abuse from a different perspective: think about your best friend for just a few moments. How objective are you about your best friend? How often do you routinely overlook their faults and forgive your best friend? To many addicts, their drug of choice is their best friend, and they are unable to clearly see negative things about their drug while they are still actively using it.

Most forms of substance abuse are associated with higher rates of depression. Research shows that the rates of depression are *double* in those who vape nicotine.[7] Also, research has long shown that smoking cigarettes is associated with higher rates of depression.[8]

Actively using/abusing substances can make it very hard to benefit from antidepressant medication. Regardless of the substance, I strongly recommend sobriety in the treatment of depression.

Medication Treatments Can and Do Save Lives in Depression

While it makes sense to have an awareness of the limitations of antidepressants, it is also important to recognize that antidepressants can be very helpful in the treatment of depression. You can also consider genetic testing to potentially improve the odds of effectiveness and reduce the chance of side effects of medications. New medications are being researched in order to find even more effective treatments for depression. To increase your chances of responding to treatment, consider if you need to reduce or stop using alcohol and other drugs.

Reflection

- Read Proverbs 15:22. Do you believe the counsel in the verse could apply to receiving counseling about medications? Why or why not?

- If you had depression, would you consider taking an antidepressant? Why or why not?

7. Obisesan et al., "E-Cigarette Use and Depression," 3–7.
8. Boden et al., "Smoking and Depression," 443–45.

- If you would not feel comfortable taking an antidepressant, would doing some genetic testing increase your confidence in doing so?

- If you had depression, would you be more likely to try a traditional antidepressant, something like prescribed ketamine, or an investigational medication? Why?

- What are your thoughts about the medical data on the effects of cannabis and alcohol on depression?

- Are there any steps that you plan to take as a result of reading this chapter (for example, sharing this information with others, considering an antidepressant if you avoided it in the past, or reducing/eliminating cannabis or alcohol use)?

9

Brain Stimulation for Stubborn or Severe Depression

For the Spirit God gave us does not make us timid, but gives us power, love and self-discipline. (2 Timothy 1:7)

What Do You Do When Nothing Seems to Work for Your Depression?

I'M A PSYCHIATRIST AND I'm faced with this question every day in my clinical practice. What can be done for patients when traditional treatment approaches aren't working?

I have worked with many severely and chronically depressed people who have tried a range of medications and worked with several therapists but have never found lasting relief. This is demoralizing for patients and for the people trying to help them.

One of the challenges in these situations is that the depressed person may be unable, unwilling, or unconvinced to do the daily behaviors, such as exercise, behavioral activation, and psychotherapy, that would help pull them out of the depression. In a way, they need a break from their depression symptoms so that they actually have the motivation, willingness, and energy to start doing those healthy things that will help them escape their depression.

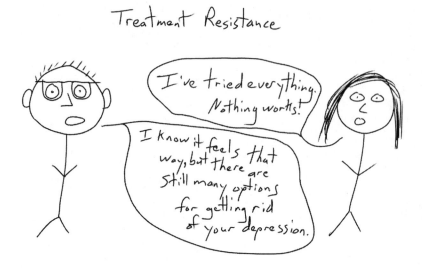

When medications and therapy aren't working, the two non-medication treatments that have shown the most promise for treatment-resistant depression are electroconvulsive therapy (ECT) and transcranial magnetic stimulation (TMS). ECT and TMS can be the breakthrough that some depressed people need. I'll describe both treatments in detail below. However, I first want to share with you a personal story from my clinical practice.

Changing One Thing Changed Everything

My wife Krista (who is also a psychiatrist) and I moved to Montana after completing our medical training because we wanted to use our skills in an area with high needs. Montana is a large, rural state with a population of one million people. It also happens to have one of the highest suicide rates in the nation. Krista and I worked for ten years for an agency that serves children and adults with severe mental illness and developmental disabilities before transitioning to our private practice.

In our private practice, we began to see more and more people with severe, chronic depression. Despite having severe depression, many of these people were still doing everything possible to take care of their families and hold down one or more jobs. Our hearts were with them as we worked to find solutions for their depression. We tried many different antidepressants, used researched-backed strategies for medication combinations, and worked in a coordinated manner with their therapists, many of whom were exceptional. We even convinced a substantial portion of our patients to exercise and engage in behavioral activation strategies. Unfortunately, some of these patients still did not get better.

An additional challenge that we faced was that many of our depressed patients firmly refused to pursue electroconvulsive therapy (ECT), which is considered to be the gold standard intervention for treatment-resistant depression but was not available in our community. Our patients were refusing ECT due to stigma, cost, lack of availability, and side effects. We were aware of the emerging treatments of ketamine therapy and transcranial magnetic stimulation (TMS) and decided that we wanted to have more options available for our patients and the community. After reviewing the research, we began to consider adding TMS to our outpatient practice.

We prayed a great deal over the decision. It was a big step, and God gave us the conviction to move forward with TMS. We believed that God wanted us to do it and that he would provide for us. We obtained additional training and certification and changed nearly everything in our clinical practice. We moved our practice to obtain more space, purchased a TMS machine, and nearly tripled our staff to accommodate the new treatment. We also had to figure out a way to spread the word about the treatment to our own patients and the community.

TMS was approved by the FDA for the treatment of depression in 2008, but many people have never heard of it or developed any trust that it will work. Using magnetic pulses to cure depression may sound like pseudoscience, but studies show its effectiveness for treatment-resistant depression. Half the patients we have treated with TMS have reached remission (full freedom) of their depression. In total, 75 percent of our TMS patients achieve a meaningful clinical response. Some of the people who have benefited from TMS and achieved remission or response had experienced enormous trauma in their lives and been depressed for decades, yet TMS therapy still worked for them.

Krista and I have made several sacrifices to provide TMS in our small town, but it has been worth it. God has provided for us so that we can provide for others. Many of the patients we previously had been unable to help are now free from depression, and some of them are also free from medication.

Electroconvulsive Therapy (ECT) for Depression

While I believe that TMS is the direction neuroscience is going in finding ever-better treatments for severe depression, it is important to acknowledge that ECT is currently considered to be the gold standard intervention for treatment-resistant depression. A medical review found that ECT has remission rates of 70 to 90 percent in clinical trials but lower remission rates (30 to 47 percent) in real-life, community studies.[1] While the mechanism by which ECT works is not fully understood, it is hypothesized that ECT enhances neuroplasticity, which allows depressed people to form new, non-depressed neural connections in their brains.

ECT, which has sometimes been referred to as "shock therapy," has unfortunately been portrayed by Hollywood and the media as a form of abuse or punishment. Nothing could be further from the truth! The physicians who provide ECT are doing a tremendous service for patients and communities. ECT's benefit is often rapid, and it saves lives; however, it can be hard to convince people of that if they have seen movies such as *One Flew Over the Cuckoo's Nest*, which inaccurately portrays ECT as punishment and torture rather than a healing treatment performed under anesthesia.

The way ECT is performed is that the person receiving treatment is placed under general anesthesia, given a medication that temporarily paralyzes muscles, and then a brief seizure is initiated with electricity. The person receiving ECT is unconscious during the process, not in pain, and remains still throughout the procedure. The reality of ECT treatment is that it is a calm medical procedure performed by a team of professionals.

Most people who receive ECT have six to twelve treatments over the course of several weeks. After each treatment, people are often confused for minutes to hours as they are recovering both from general anesthesia and the seizure. It is common for people to experience temporary memory loss, and some people, unfortunately, experience some degree of permanent memory loss. Most of my patients who chose not to pursue ECT did so because of three factors: availability (it is harder to access as it is not available in our community), cost (ECT costs about twice as much as TMS), and the risk of memory impairment. I am certainly not against ECT, as I have seen it cure people's depression, and if I have a patient with extremely severe depression or who has not responded to TMS, I often recommend

---

1. Prudic et al., "Electroconvulsive Therapy," 304–10.

that they pursue ECT. ECT has been proven over decades to be effective both for major depression and bipolar depression.

ECT	TMS
The gold standard for resistant depression	Very effective for resistant depression
Involves the generation of a seizure	No seizure
Relies on electricity	Relies on magnetic pulses
Involves anesthesia	No anesthesia

Transcranial Magnetic Stimulation (TMS) Therapy for Depression

You may remember from chapters 2 and 3 that there are unique changes that occur in the depressed brain. In addition to changes in brain region activity, such as decreased activity in the left frontal lobe, there is also an overall decrease in communication between the frontal lobe (thinking center) and limbic system (emotional center).

In TMS therapy, we stimulate the frontal lobe to get the regions of the brain communicating with each other normally again. TMS therapy utilizes powerful repetitive magnetic pulses that stimulate the left frontal lobe as well as neural pathways/circuits that are underactive in individuals with depression. The magnetic pulses actually stimulate, or depolarize, neurons in the brain. By activating the underactive networks in a depressed brain, TMS repeatedly stimulates pathways of the brain to "talk" to each other. It is as though we are telling the brain, "This is what you gotta do . . . this is what you gotta do . . ." over and over until the brain does it on its own.

Different medical offices run different protocols when they deliver TMS therapy. For example, some clinics might treat for three to six minutes every day over six weeks or less. At our office, the person will arrive at the same time each day for a twenty-minute treatment Monday through Friday for six weeks. The treatment is then tapered to three days of treatment in week seven, two days of treatment in week eight, and the final treatment in week nine. Patients also are encouraged to meet weekly with their therapist, exercise regularly, and maintain a consistent sleep schedule. To decrease the risk of seizure (a rare side effect of TMS) and to enhance responsiveness to TMS, the patient is expected to abstain from alcohol and other recreational drugs throughout their treatment course.

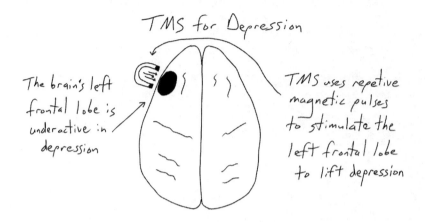

TMS for Depression

The brain's left frontal lobe is underactive in depression

TMS uses repetive magnetic pulses to stimulate the left frontal lobe to lift depression

The FDA has approved TMS for the treatment of moderate to severe major depression after one unsuccessful antidepressant trial in adults age twenty-two to seventy. Most private insurance companies and Medicare pay for TMS treatment for people age eighteen and older, but many insurance companies set higher requirements (such as more medication and therapy trials) before they will cover the treatment. While there is research demonstrating that TMS therapy is safe and effective for kids, it is harder to get insurance companies to cover the treatment for people under age eighteen.[2]

One of the benefits of TMS therapy is that it has relatively few side effects. Most TMS side effects diminish and resolve after the first week of treatment. Side effects may include headache, treatment site discomfort, and jaw discomfort. There is also a rare risk of seizure (3/50,000 treatments) which is comparable to or lower than some psychiatric medications. For example, the seizure risk of the antidepressant Wellbutrin (bupropion) is higher, at about 250/50,000 patients. There are no systemic or sexual side effects to TMS therapy, as contrasted with many antidepressant medications.

TMS therapy does not require psychiatric medication to work. It works when traditional treatments such as medication and therapy aren't working. TMS therapy is FDA approved, and scientific research proves that it works with comparable efficacy to ECT. When comparing the two treatments, many patients choose TMS therapy for reasons such as:

- No anesthesia is involved.

2. Wall et al., "Neurocognitive Effects," 3–6.

- People can drive themselves to/from their treatment.
- No seizure is involved.
- No memory impairment occurs.
- People can return to work right after each treatment.
- The treatment time is shorter (usually twenty minutes or less).
- The cost is lower.
- There are more treatment centers available.

Other Aspects of TMS Therapy

TMS therapy does not just benefit a person during their treatment course. Among the people who achieve remission (full freedom from depression) or response (depressive symptoms are cut in half), about two-thirds of those people will maintain their level of improvement at least a full year later.[3] When the treatment works, the benefit tends to stick. Additionally, if TMS therapy is needed again in the future, the treatment is likely to work again.[4]

There are factors in treatment that affect the outcome. One is having a friendly technician who runs the treatment. Another factor is directed thoughts. In one study,[5] positively directed and neutral thoughts during TMS therapy sessions resulted in better outcomes than negatively directed thoughts. We use this medical research in our clinic to improve outcomes. You may recall when I described balancing thoughts (cognitive reframing) and using biblical affirmations to counter negative thoughts in chapter 3. We help our patients to get into a better mental state during treatment to improve outcomes. Some of our patients choose to bring in Bible verses that are special to them and that they can reflect on during treatment.

Recent Developments in TMS

There is something new being studied in TMS therapy: treating many times per day over a shorter timeframe. In Stanford's SAINT (Stanford Accelerated Intelligent Neuromodulation Therapy) study, Dr. Nolan Williams

3. Dunner et al., "Multisite, Naturalistic, Observational Study," 1397–99.
4. Kelly et al., "Initial Response," 180–81.
5. Isserles et al., "Cognitive–Emotional Reactivation," 238–41.

and his research team gave patients fifty TMS treatments over five days and achieved a 90.5 percent remission rate. However, they only followed patients for five weeks after treatment, so it's not known how long the improvement lasts.[6] The world is looking at this small study and how Stanford arranged their treatment procedures to see if this is the best new treatment for depression using TMS. Stanford's SAINT protocol:

- Gives more TMS treatments.

- Shortens the treatment to five days.

- May have superior outcomes.

- Allows easier access to people from rural areas.

- Might become the new gold standard for resistant depression.

The SAINT study protocol is not ready for widespread clinical application, but the science behind it appears sound. In 2022, this same Stanford team published results of another small SAINT study that included a placebo, and depressed people who received the treatment achieved a 79 percent remission rate.[7] The researchers also renamed the approach Stanford Neuromodulation Therapy (SNT). These are small studies that need to be replicated. If larger studies find similar results, it could be a complete game-changer in terms of how all TMS is delivered. Imagine a future in which five days of intense treatment could reverse decades of depression. It's exciting that a new TMS treatment protocol could nearly double the chances of remission of depression. Time will tell if these studies will hold up. If they do, it will be transformative for our families and communities, and it might just become the new gold standard intervention for treatment-resistant depression.

Why Not Just Skip Medication and Start Treatment with TMS Therapy?

I hear this a lot from people: "If TMS therapy is so effective and it has relatively few side effects, why not just start with TMS therapy?" I think this is a great question. One of the challenges of accessing TMS therapy is that, even though the cost is roughly half that of ECT, it is still expensive. Any medical

---

6. Cole et al., "Stanford Accelerated," 720–24.
7. Cole et al., "Stanford Neuromodulation Therapy," 134–37.

intervention that takes thirty-six treatments is going to be costly due to the multiplier effect (36 x $100 = $3,600; 36 x $200 = $7,200; etc.). The SAINT/SNT protocol requires even more, with fifty total treatments.

If a medical treatment will take a person to their individual out-of-pocket maximum limit for their health insurance, that person might want a guarantee that the treatment will work, but the best TMS outcomes to date (excluding the small SAINT and SNT studies) have a remission rate of around 50 percent. The cost of Prozac (fluoxetine) is a few cents per pill and it works amazingly well in treating many people's depression, so it is usually recommended to start with an antidepressant medication.

Also, even though TMS therapy treatment only takes minutes per day, it needs to be performed in a medical clinic, not at home, so treatment involves scheduling time to travel to/from appointments and time for the TMS therapy session. It takes effort for patients to build TMS therapy into their daily schedule. Many people prefer the convenience of taking an anti-depressant medication as long as they find it to be effective, affordable, and to have minimal side effects.

TMS Therapy and ECT Are Two Powerful Treatments That Work When Others Have Failed

It's important to know what your options are when treating depression. There are even more (less commonly known or utilized) depression treatments that I have not covered in this book. Sometimes people believe they have tried everything only to learn that there are more options to consider. It gives them hope to know that more strategies can be tried until they achieve full freedom from depression. The field of medicine is continuing to develop more effective treatments for depression that directly target brain circuitry that is not working normally in the depressed brain. There is realistic hope that there will be faster, less costly, and even more effective treatments in the future.

Reflection

- Read 2 Timothy 1:7. What does this verse make you think about? How do you see this verse speaking to the concept of courage?

- If you had extreme depression that didn't respond to medication and therapy, would you consider ECT? Why or why not?

- If you had treatment-resistant depression and had to choose between ECT and TMS, which would you choose? Why?

- What is your reaction to hearing about the outcomes of the SAINT and SNT studies? Does this give you hope in any way?

- What do you think about cost considerations when choosing a depression treatment?

- Are there any steps that you plan to take as a result of reading this chapter (for example, sharing this information with someone you know who is depressed and discouraged)?

III

The Journey to Health

Getting Better, Staying Better, and Helping Others

10

Tools and Strategies

"For I know the plans I have for you," declares the Lord,
"Plans to prosper you and not to harm you, plans to
give you hope and a future." (Jeremiah 29:11)

Strategies for Getting Better and Staying Better.

THIS FINAL SECTION OF the book is about getting to full freedom from depression and staying there, especially if some of your original strategies for your depression were not effective. One of the most frustrating aspects of depression is that it leaves people feeling helpless and thinking, "There's nothing I can do to fix this!" I want you to know that you have many options to get your mood better and for the treatments that you use for depression to be as effective as possible.

This chapter is about *strategies* and *tools*. Having a good overall plan with the right strategies for using effective tools will give you the best odds of getting fully free from depression, especially if your depression is treatment resistant. Your tools might include:

- Mood-rating scales.
- A written treatment plan.

- A written safety plan.

- A log of past treatment.

- A book that reminds you how to replace negative thoughts with balanced thoughts.

A Plan Is Better than No Plan

When the first thing you try for your depression works, then having a plan centered on the treatment of your mood seems unnecessary. But what would you do if the first treatment didn't work or the depression came back? It's at this point that setting up a plan that is unique to you is critical in getting to remission.

Using a few tools is not the same as actually having a plan. Following a plan, not just trying random tools, is important not only in depression treatment but also in many areas of life. I've spoken to many people who have struggled for years and "tried meds" or "tried therapy" only to find that their depression never fully improved. To be fair, some people have not been told all of their options for depression treatment. In other cases, because of their depression, they have low motivation and energy, which block them from following the recommended steps.

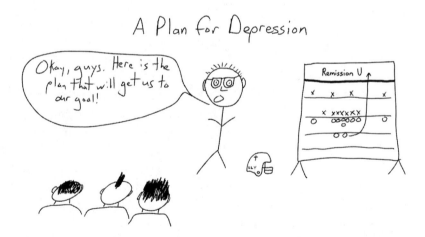

A treatment plan in psychiatry involves setting measurable goals and regularly checking in on the progress toward those goals. I like treatment plans, especially when they are unique, relevant to the individual, and regularly reviewed. The challenge that I have seen with many treatment plans over time is that they all look the same, have generic recommendations, and are ignored after they are created.

Another difficulty I see with some treatment plans is that they do not set the bar high enough. For example, in the treatment of depression, I am not satisfied unless someone achieves full remission of their depression and can stay depression-free. Do you want to feel only partially better or do you want to be cured of your depression? If you want a cure, are you willing to do what is necessary to get there? In treating depression, I like to think about a comprehensive plan, specific to the individual, that involves strategies with a high likelihood of helping.

Here is an example of a treatment plan that I might help set up for the unique needs of one of my patients (please keep in mind that not everything listed is equally effective):

1. *Therapy*: Goal—meet weekly with my therapist.

2. *Psychiatry*: Goal—meet every two to four weeks with my psychiatrist if I'm struggling (every six to twelve weeks if I'm doing better).

3. *Spiritual*: Goal—attend my weekly prayer group (or Bible study).

4. *Exercise*: Goal—get to the gym (intention: three days per week) and increase total physical activity, such as walking at lunch (intention: five days per week).

5. *Positive activity*: Goal—select and do at least one behavioral activation strategy from my list daily.

6. *Sobriety*: Goal—abstain from alcohol.

7. *Diet*: Goal—eat regular meals and only one fast food meal per week.

8. *Sleep*: Goal—get myself in bed by 11 p.m. with the target of sleeping seven to nine hours.

9. *Social media*: Goal—limit my time on social media to a maximum of thirty minutes per day, three times per week.

10. *Safety*: Goal—review the adequacy of my safety plan at each therapy and psychiatry visit and make changes if anything on the plan is ineffective.

It is helpful to keep a log so that you can record your progress and be accountable to yourself. There is nothing magic about this plan or the number ten. There may be dozens of elements to a good depression plan, but the higher the number, the more overwhelming it can feel to a person who is already struggling with low motivation and energy.

Rating Scales Can Inspire Action, Document Progress, and Catch Safety Problems

While at the end of the day you either have depression or you don't, if you are not measuring your depression, you could be missing out on the opportunity to document your progress, something that would motivate you and your doctor in your journey to freedom from depression. Also, measuring your depression helps clarify if your treatment plan is working or needs changing.

Consider a different illness, such as diabetes. Imagine trying to get quality treatment for your diabetes if you were unable to measure your blood sugar or other signs of the condition. How would that even work? I suppose you would meet with your endocrinologist every few weeks. Your endocrinologist might ask you questions about your diet such as, "And when you ate that doughnut, how did that make you feel?" Your endocrinologist might then suggest that you exercise more and that a different medication might help. While this example may seem ridiculous, it shows the absurdity of treating an illness without enough data.

Now, consider depression. Many people receive treatment for their depression with therapy and antidepressants, yet there are no widely available biological measures, or biomarkers, of depression as there are for diabetes. One of the closest tools to biomarkers for depression is rating scales. Depression rating scales are formal tests or measures of your mood in which you answer questions about various problems that are common in depression. Based on your answers, you can learn more about whether you might have major depression and how severe the depression is. Rating scales alone do not diagnose depression, as only your doctor or therapist can make the diagnosis. However, depression rating scales can assist in:

- Confirming a depression diagnosis.
- Opening up conversations for dealing with depression.
- Measuring your progress.
- Accessing and implementing more intensive, effective treatments.

- Improving the understanding of your doctor and therapist about what you are going through. This is especially important if you frequently say that you feel "fine" when:

  - You aren't fine at all.

  - You don't want to deal with the other person's reaction.

  - You don't want to hurt your doctor's or therapist's feelings if you aren't getting better.

  - You are not dialed in to how you feel.

  - You feel better than you used to but are still struggling.

  - You don't want your doctor to change your medication.

A commonly used depression rating scale is the Patient Health Questionnaire (PHQ-9). This depression screening tool is self-administered, well-validated, and short (it has only ten questions and usually takes less than three minutes to complete). The PHQ-9 is used to screen for depression, assist in its diagnosis, and track symptoms over the course of treatment. It has other benefits, such as being free to use/reproduce, and is widely used in primary care settings. The only downside I have seen with the PHQ-9 is that it does not capture the true severity of depression for some patients. When I suspect this is occurring, I have those patients complete different depression rating scales.

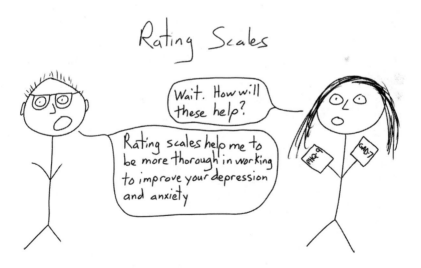

Millions of people in the US have received treatment and achieved freedom from depression after never having completed a depression rating scale. So why bother with them? There are many reasons for using depression rating scales, including:

- Research shows that the faster you achieve remission (full freedom from depression), the more likely you are to stay in remission.
- If you settle for just being partially better rather than seeking full remission, it can set you up for chronic or recurring depression.
- Your doctor or therapist may have no clue how bad your depression is or how much you are suffering.
- You may have limited awareness of the severity of your depression until you use a standard measure.
- The use of depression rating scales adds a greater degree of objectivity to an otherwise subjective assessment process.
- In medicine, things that are measured are things that can be improved.

It can also be helpful to complete the Generalized Anxiety Disorder 7-item scale (GAD-7). It can be helpful to monitor how your anxiety and depression change relative to each other, and it can provide an opportunity for you to address your anxiety if it is elevated (elevated anxiety can trigger depression).

Completing rating scales is your opportunity to provide honest feedback to your psychiatrist and therapist. Their response to your completed scale may provide you with the information you need about what to do next in your treatment, especially if your goal is to achieve full freedom from depression.

You can review the PHQ-9 and the GAD-7 in the "Resources" section. They are free to use and copy.

Record Keeping Is Necessary

For most people, keeping an updated list of every medication they have ever tried for depression is the most boring and tedious thing in the world, especially if they are already depressed. It can also be really hard to go back years or decades and try to figure out the names of all the therapists you saw and the medications you tried.

You might think that your medical records will always be there, but unfortunately that is not always the case. All states have laws that require medical records for adults from the past five to ten years to be available (there are a few exceptions in certain states) and for medical records to be available for a slightly longer period for children. Federal law requires a similar range for medical record retention for certain health insurance plans.

Most people are disturbed to learn that their six-year-old medical records might be gone. This can create a huge problem for patients, especially because insurance companies, when covering a more expensive treatment, often require evidence that a less expensive medication/intervention was previously tried and failed. Even if you have used the same pharmacy for decades, you might have a very hard time getting your past prescription records that are more than a year old. Pharmacies, hospitals, and clinics update their software frequently, and when they do this, there can be problems accessing older records that were created by previous software.

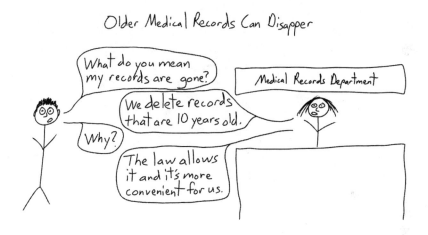

Older Medical Records Can Disapper

There are options. Most of the strategies involve active effort on your part. You have a right to access your medical records and can request copies. The 21st Century Cures Act allows people to have free electronic access to their medical records at most facilities. Other requests for medical records, such as paper copies or faxes, often involve a fee.

You might consider keeping your own summary of treatment. This is not a bad idea, as most electronic medical records systems in the US do not communicate with each other. Until that changes in our country, you might be the best person to keep track of your past and current medical treatments.

The information that can be helpful in treating your depression is extensive and might require a lot of effort to collect. Please don't get demoralized if you choose to do this. You might feel like giving up when you look at your list of unsuccessful treatments. A skilled psychiatrist might look at the same list and wonder why you have not tried a dozen other strategies. Information that can be helpful includes:

- A detailed list of medications (including dates and dosages).
- Therapist names and dates and types of therapy.
- Assessments and evaluations performed.
- Hospitalizations and placements.
- Interventions like transcranial magnetic stimulation (TMS) therapy, electroconvulsive therapy (ECT), and ketamine/esketamine.
- Other strategies you have tried or are currently utilizing.

In the hands of a knowledgeable psychiatrist, a record of past treatment yields critical information. Good psychiatric care starts with an accurate diagnosis, and sometimes a clear record of the failure of multiple appropriate medications leads to a review and revision of a diagnosis, resulting in more effective treatment. Additionally, information about all your past treatments for depression can help you and your doctor to:

- Return to the treatment that worked best.
- Discover errors in medication treatment.
- Prevent a retrial of a medication that didn't work or led to an adverse reaction.
- Discover diagnostic errors.
- Address treatment nonadherence.
- Uncover nonmedical interventions that you didn't know were effective.
- Obtain pharmacogenetic testing.
- Try a treatment that you didn't initially consider.
- Document the severity of the illness to show medical necessity for more expensive treatments.

A final note on putting together a treatment record is that it can help you deal with avoidance. Some people use every possible strategy, yet still struggle with depression. However, others with treatment-resistant depression show a clear pattern of avoidance and continually skip doses of their medications and/or effective interventions such as psychotherapy, behavioral activation, and exercise.

Bibliotherapy

Bibliotherapy for depression is the act of reading a book that has been shown to help depression. One of the best known of these books is *Feeling Good* by Dr. David Burns. Research has shown substantial benefits from bibliotherapy.[1] Some of the most beneficial books help people to clearly see how their thoughts shape their emotions, and by replacing unbalanced thoughts with more balanced ones, people can experience improvement in their depression.

Something as simple as giving the book *Feeling Good* to a depressed person could provide lasting benefit *if they read it and follow its instructions.*[2] One of the nice aspects of having a book is the ability to go back and reference helpful sections if you struggle with your mood in the future. While giving a depressed person the book *unJoy* may be helpful as bibliotherapy, it has not yet been researched as bibliotherapy.

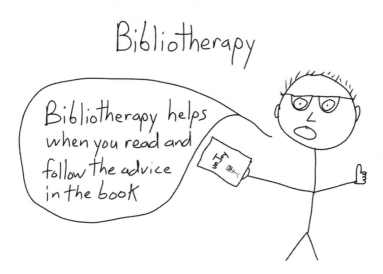

1. Gregory et al., "Bibliotherapy for Depression," 277–79.
2. Smith et al., "Three-Year Follow-Up," 325–26.

Hospital-Based Treatments

You might be surprised to see hospital-based treatments in my tools and strategies chapter; however, a temporary intervention in the hospital could be the difference between life and death when it comes to suicide risk and other health risks when struggling with depression.

If you are unable to maintain your safety or basic functioning (sleeping, eating, hygiene), you might need to consider a brief stay in a hospital setting until your mood, safety, and functioning improve. Some of the most common hospital-based treatments are:

- Acute psychiatric hospitalization: This treatment involves checking into the hospital's psychiatric program for a few days to up to a couple of weeks.

- Partial hospitalization programs: This treatment involves the structured treatment you could receive at an acute program, but you travel each day to the hospital for treatment rather than remaining continuously at the hospital.

- Residential treatment programs: This treatment involves checking into a program and staying there for weeks to months to work on a specific issue, such as addressing recurrent suicidal thoughts, learning/practicing coping skills, or having more time to improve your depression.

Strategies and Tools for Getting Better, Faster

If you are struggling with depression, it is important to know what treatments and tools are available and to have an overall plan of action. Using the tools and strategies in this chapter will help you access a variety of treatments more systematically and effectively. In addition to this book, there are other books you can read and reference that can help you when you are depressed. And if you know someone who is struggling, you can share all of these resources with them as well.

Reflection

- Read Jeremiah 29:11. In what ways are you encouraged by what God is saying in this verse?

- Do you believe that a proactive plan for treating depression is likely to yield better results? Why or why not?

- What are your thoughts about completing rating scales and keeping a record of past successes and ineffective treatments? Do you think it would be helpful or demoralizing? Is this worth doing?

- Do you believe a nonreligious book can be helpful to Christians who have depression? Why or why not?

- Are there any steps that you plan to take as a result of reading this chapter (for example, using rating scales, checking out the book *Feeling Good*, creating a treatment plan, or sharing some of this information with a loved one with depression)?

11

Preparing Yourself for Positive Change

But those who hope in the Lord will renew their strength.
They will soar on wings like eagles; they will run and not grow
weary, they will walk and not be faint. (Isaiah 40:31)

The Secret Fear of Getting Better

I'VE HEARD VERY FEW experts talk about the secret fear that many chronically depressed people have about getting free from their depression. Addressing this issue is critical for many people with treatment-resistant depression because these fears can block improvement.

Many depressed people have substantial difficulty in shifting their perspective from their current situation. They cannot correctly imagine how their lives and functioning will be when they are finally free from depression. Instead of imagining happiness, energy, motivation, and joy, they can only imagine that they will still feel the way they currently do but that others' expectations of them will increase. For example, they may say to themselves, "My biggest accomplishment today was getting out of bed and brushing my teeth. Afterward, I was completely exhausted. I can't imagine feeling this way and being expected to work forty hours each week. I'll just end up failing and that will make me feel even more depressed." Because the desired outcome is feared, the depressed person may consciously or unconsciously resist behavioral changes that could lead to improvement. If the secret fear of getting better is not addressed, a person might not be able to get their depression better, even if a part of them wanted to.

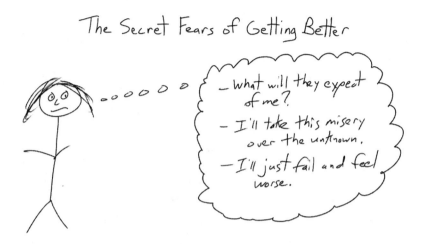

People sometimes wish for contradictory outcomes in depression: feeling better but not changing a thing in their lives. Do you see the problem with this thinking? If these contradictions are not resolved, they will interfere with the improvement of depression. Sticking with behaviors and patterns you have when depressed can prevent recovery from depression.

I May Be in a Rut, but It's My Rut

Most people are drawn to what is familiar and comfortable. They have a favorite meal at a favorite restaurant. They have a favorite set of clothes that they like to lounge in at home. There can be tremendous comfort in doing familiar things. The longer you do them, the harder change can be.

This is also true regarding depression. Some people have been depressed for so long that their depression becomes their constant and main companion. Spending time with friends and involving themselves in other activities may have gone by the wayside long ago. They are stuck in the rut of depression, but it's a really comfortable rut. If this sounds like you, you might be wondering, "If my depression was gone, what would I do with my life?" Not having a good answer to that question can interfere with getting better.

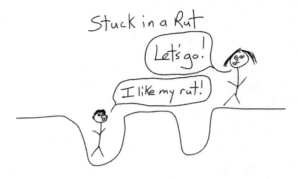

Behavioral activation strategies can help with this dilemma, and you can do them even when you are depressed. Activities that are in alignment with your values can feel like a safe way to pull yourself out of the comfort zone of depression.

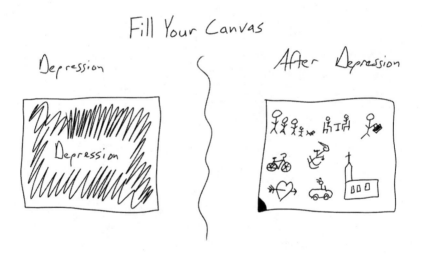

The life canvas on the right is filled with activities, and the depression is compressed down into the bottom left corner of the canvas. Not filling your life with activities will invite the depression to return and expand to fill your canvas again.

Consider looking at all the things you do in your life and how those activities might be pictured on an art canvas. When you are depressed, the entire canvas is often filled by the depression. If you had no other activities and the depression magically disappeared, your life canvas might look pretty blank, which is anxiety-provoking. While depression itself can feel familiar and comfortable, consider adding in some safe discomfort to start filling your life canvas with positive activities. Even if you could snap your fingers and get rid of your depression, a blank canvas would be an invitation for the depression to return. Both when getting rid of depression and after achieving full freedom from depression, it is important to have a life filled with activities that align with your values.

Most People Don't Want to Be "Fixed"

One of the challenges in getting depression better is the fear of losing something that you value about yourself. You might worry that someone is trying to take away authentic emotional reactions that fuel your creativity, such as in your writing, art, or music. Or you might worry that someone is trying to change your personality.

I can think of many people who would not want to improve their depression if they feared it would steal something they value about themselves. These fears need to be addressed, and working with a skilled therapist can help you to effectively do so. In therapy, consider spending as much time as you need to review and acknowledge what you value about yourself *before* jumping to possible solutions.

Depression That Is Self-punishment

There is a small percentage of Christians whose depression is a form of self-punishment that interferes in their healing from depression. For them, they may believe it is their duty to show God how badly they feel about their past behavior by experiencing misery as a means of atonement or penance. If this sounds like you, I want you to know that you cannot atone for your past but can receive forgiveness and freedom from your past through Jesus. He is our atonement. God does not desire your misery. Yes, God calls upon Christians to endure suffering, but he does not command us to bring suffering on ourselves unnecessarily. God sent us the precious gift of Jesus to free us from guilt, shame, and regret. God does not call us to wallow in self-pity or past regrets. Jesus said, "I have come that they may have life, and have it to the full" (John 10:10).

Dealing with Depression Can Involve Some Uncomfortable Truths

When you get free from depression, you might be forced to deal with things you had previously avoided. Some people can become so focused on climbing out of their depression that they become overwhelmed when they see other problems in their lives, problems that were previously obscured by the fog of their depression.

Depression may have kept a person from working, sometimes for decades. If they get free from depression, does that mean they are immediately ready to reenter the workforce? People can be faced with other challenges when depression no longer robs them of energy. What if you become free from depression and see more clearly that:

- Your kids are drifting away or spiraling out of control.

- You have to deal with difficulties in your marriage.

- You might need to change jobs.

What are you going to do with a non-depressed life? I've seen people make some incredible changes as they have become free of depression, including switching jobs, ending unhealthy long-term relationships, and moving to new towns.

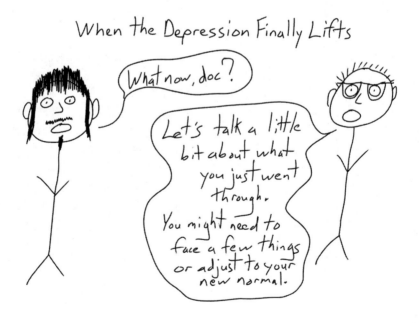

Something else to prepare for when you improve your depression is that other emotions might rise to the surface, in particular irritability and anxiety. It's not uncommon that people's anxiety and irritability are lower when they are severely depressed because they stop caring about things they normally care about. In a way, they feel emotionally numb. When the depression lifts, they feel less numb and start caring again, or they begin to have the energy to take action in areas they cared about all along.

When people finally get free from prolonged, severe depression, they might worry that they are undergoing a personality change as their anxiety and irritability increase. This is not the case. However, when their depression lifts, people often have to start managing other emotions.

A Story about Moving Past Resistance to Improvement

Janie was a forty-five-year-old woman who had been depressed for five years. Her depression started when she was laid off from work during an economic recession; however, she never made it back into the workforce. Janie had been depressed for so long, it felt like it had become her new normal. All of the doctors and therapists that she met with annoyed her as they all had solutions—medications or therapy techniques—that they wanted her to try without first getting to know her and her unique situation.

She had met with several therapists, but her new one was different. Something interesting happened in her first session. Her therapist, Andy, listened without interruption to her long list of failed strategies. She finished telling her therapist about her experience with a strong statement that nothing would work and this was just her life now.

Janie was feeling a little anxious as she told her story because she kept expecting to be interrupted. So many of her previous doctors interrupted her and offered solutions before they truly listened to her. The most powerful thing Andy did in that first session was that he didn't try to fix her. Andy's "doing nothing" except listening and showing empathy helped her lower her guard a bit.

At the end of the first session, Andy said, "I think I can help you. I think you are stuck in your depression exactly how you described it. If you want to work with me, we'll find out why. We'll look at the positive and negative sides of everything that you think and do that influences your depression. In the end, we'll figure out what steps, if any, you are willing to take to get out of this depression. There is a cost to getting better. You'll be the judge who determines if it's worth it. Something I can tell you, though, is that you will not have to give up the things you value about yourself to do it."

Janie worked in therapy with Andy for a year. He had this interesting way of getting her to challenge herself on what she said she wanted in life and to prove to herself that she really wanted it. Because he understood her perspective, he was able to help her to reframe some of her maladaptive thoughts by seeing how these actually misrepresented her core values. He gave her strategies to trick herself into doing healthy activities that her depression told her were impossible. Through her work in therapy, Janie concluded that she truly wanted the depression to end and she knew what it would cost her. It took time, but she eventually was able to get free from her depression. While it was hard work and it was uncomfortable at times recovering from depression, Janie expanded her life to include many activities and more time with friends and family, and she eventually reentered the workforce on a part-time basis.

Work with a Professional When You Are Pulling Out of Serious Depression

Working with a skilled therapist can make all the difference in the world as you strive to rid yourself of depression. This is especially true if you have been depressed for a very long time. I've worked to help patients who have been depressed for decades finally become 100 percent free from depression. The depression had changed their lives so dramatically that after recovering, they felt a bit adrift. In their depression, they had given up on numerous activities and relationships. They may have resigned themselves to being single or pulled back emotionally from others as they felt utterly undesirable in their depression.

A skilled therapist can help you work through considering what life pursuits you plan to go after when you are free of depression. They can also help you in the grief process. This might sound a bit strange, but many people who have been depressed for a prolonged time go through a period of grief *for themselves* after they have recovered from depression and feel it is safe to revisit that dark time in their lives. Working with a professional who understands this grief and can help you see it as a normal part of the healing process can be very validating and encouraging as you close the depression chapter of your life and begin the next.

Knowing the Risks Will Help You

Feeling stuck in depression is demoralizing. While there might be steps that you can take to get out of the depression, taking those steps and doing them consistently can feel impossible. Also, some treatments may seem artificial or even threatening if they don't take into account what makes your situation unique or the things that you value about yourself. There are solutions when you are stuck and feeling resigned to your situation or confused and anxious about what to do next. Filling your life canvas with activities that are in alignment with your values is a great place to start. Choosing to work with a skilled therapist who gets to know you and what you value most will also help you to determine and pursue the next steps you need to take to get free from depression.

Reflection

- Read Isaiah 40:31. What emotional reaction do you have reading this verse? Does it give you hope in any way?
- Can you see how getting better could potentially seem terrifying to someone who is very depressed?
- What do you think about the assertion that getting out of depression could increase irritability or anxiety?
- Are there any steps that you plan to take as a result of reading this chapter (for example, mentally preparing for positive or unexpected changes in your loved one as their depression improves or praying for the courage to face a depression-free life or for guidance as your depression lifts)?

12

Helping Others Who Have Depression

Carry each other's burdens, and in this way you
will fulfill the law of Christ. (Galatians 6:2)

Keeping Hope for People Who Have None

I HAVE A FRIEND and colleague, Dr. Celeste Pfister, who summarized the importance of what we do in psychiatry in one statement. She said, "We are the guardians of hope for those who have lost theirs." People who have depression can struggle tremendously because they do not believe anything will work. Sometimes this is due to trying a few things and being disappointed with the outcome. Other times, it is due to the person engaging in substantial self-blame, because of which they don't access treatments that really work.

This is where you come in. You can be the guardian of hope for your friends and loved ones who are depressed. You can be the person who assures them that it is not their fault that they have depression, but it is their responsibility to do something about it. You can help them recognize their chronic irritability and sadness as an illness that has many effective treatments. You might be the only person in their life who can break through their denial and speak the truth that they must take one step at a time to get better. You can help them with each step and share effective treatments with them. God may be calling you to minister to the depressed people around you.

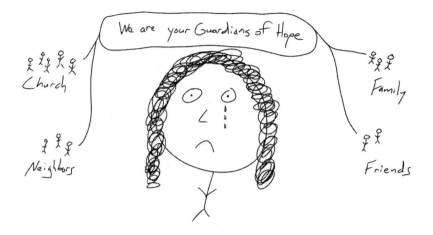

Safety Is the Best Place to Start

Helping your loved one develop an easily accessible safety plan is the first step. Make sure that you are a part of the safety plan. If your loved one is able to remain safe or notify others when they are struggling, then you have more time to implement any number of strategies. If you know someone who is depressed and is unable to maintain safety, then you may need to help them access acute psychiatric hospitalization or residential treatment. Sitting with them and ensuring they have a complete and accessible safety plan is an important step in treatment, especially for people with suicidal thoughts. Another critical component of enhancing safety is reducing access to lethal means. You can be the friend who safely stores their firearms for them until their depression is in remission and their suicidal thoughts have resolved.

IS PATH WARM?

You might wonder what common signs that signal a significant risk of suicide are. Some risk factors are considered a red flag and are captured in the acronym "IS PATH WARM?," which was created by the American Association of Suicidology. If you have lost someone to suicide, reading IS PATH WARM? can be painful. It is common for someone to think that they should have recognized all the warning signs and prevented a suicide. If you feel that way, I want to tell you not to blame yourself. You cannot predict the future. Please understand that no one, not even a psychiatrist who is trained to assess safety risk, is perfect at predicting who might attempt suicide.

Ideation—threatening to hurt or kill themselves, talking of wanting to hurt or kill themselves, or researching ways to die.

Substance abuse—excessive or increased.

Purposeless—no reasons for living, giving away important items, or finding long-term placement for pets.

Anger—intense or uncontrolled.

Trapped—feeling that there is no way out.

Hopelessness.

Withdrawal—from friends, family, and society.

Anxiety—agitation, insomnia, or too much sleep.

Recklessness—committing risky acts, seemingly without thinking.

Mood changes—dramatic.

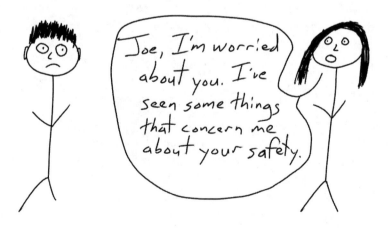

While the warning signs found in IS PATH WARM? are not the only signs that your loved one is at risk, it is important to do what is in your power to talk with them about it and take appropriate action.

Provide Them with a List of Strategies

When you start sharing with someone strategies to help their depression, be prepared to have them shoot down your ideas. Keep in mind that depression can interfere with positive memories. Sometimes people remember accurately and sometimes they forget. Do not take their insistence that something didn't work as gospel. Help them compare their report to the data and their treatment records.

It is not unusual for me to hear a patient who relapses back into depression say, "Well, I've tried everything and nothing works." Both parts of this statement are often untrue. Usually, they have not tried everything. Of the things they have tried, they have likely experienced at least a temporary or partial improvement with one or more treatments and this can shed light on a strategy that will work.

Your friend or loved one might resist your help. Be positive and persistent. I'm not suggesting that you talk them into retrying a medication that clearly didn't work or made them worse. However, sometimes people with depression avoid returning to mental health treatment due to a negative experience with a psychiatrist or psychotherapist. If that is the case, possibly one of the best things you can do is help arrange for them to see someone completely new.

What Are They Willing to Try?

There are many strategies for treating depression. Two of the most effective strategies are psychotherapy and the use of antidepressant medications. Just because a few medications were ineffective or caused side effects does not mean no medication will work. Regarding therapy, there are many evidence-based therapies to choose from in the treatment of depression. If a previous approach was ineffective, it is possible to find a different one that will resonate better with your loved one.

I've written over two dozen articles on strategies and ideas for helping depression and these articles can be accessed for free at my website (lenlantz.com/unJoy). Feel free to read these articles to your friend to see what treatment method piques their interest. In addition to therapy and antidepressants, treatments that have a large positive impact on depression include daily exercise, behavioral activation strategies, transcranial magnetic stimulation (TMS) therapy, and electroconvulsive therapy (ECT). For example, with TMS therapy, I've helped people who have been depressed for decades and have tried dozens of psychiatric medications that were ineffective.

You can encourage your loved one to try things they have been avoiding. Let them know there is help and there is hope. Remind them regularly that there is always one more thing to try, and that new treatments are being developed every year. You can tell them about the amazing depression treatment emerging from the SAINT and SNT studies that I mentioned in chapter 9.

Be a Coach Who Will Not Give Up

Family and friends with depression might need you to intrude into their world and motivate them. That is the sort of thing that a coach does. A coach does not enable unhealthy behavior. Coaching can be uncomfortable and intrusive at times, but someone who is depressed requires proactive involvement from others to get better.

Check in with your friend regularly about:

- Suicidal ideation and safety planning.
- Regular attendance of therapy.
- Daily medication adherence.
- Getting out of bed, taking care of hygiene, and putting on clean clothes daily.
- Eating regular meals even if their appetite is low.
- Maintaining a regular sleep/wake schedule.
- Taking care of their non-psychiatric health needs (for example, diabetes care).

Encourage and remind your friend regularly about:

- Their importance and uniqueness.
- Your belief in their ability to get unstuck from areas in their life that drive their depression (addictions, toxic relationships, etc.).

- Daily exercise.

- Your ability and willingness to help them problem-solve potential barriers to treatment such as cost, scheduling, childcare, or transportation.

- Your willingness to advocate for them with their doctors/therapists on their progress in depression or in receiving help for other problems like anxiety or insomnia.

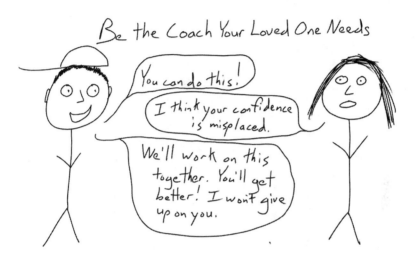

Who Can Help You?

If you are quite worried about a loved one or friend, it's best not to support them alone. Expanding the group or team of people who help will reduce your risk of burnout by sharing the load. Part of improving depression involves enlarging, not shrinking, a person's world. Decreasing isolation and expanding opportunities for human connection are incredibly powerful. The treatment team can be quite large and involve professional and natural supports.

Examples of professional supports include:

- Specialists, such as psychiatrists or psychiatric nurse practitioners.

- Psychotherapists.

- Primary care providers.

- Case managers.

- Peer supports.

Examples of natural supports include:

- Family/friends.
- Neighbors.
- Coworkers or work supervisors.
- People from a faith community.
- Mental health advocacy groups like the National Alliance on Mental Illness (NAMI).

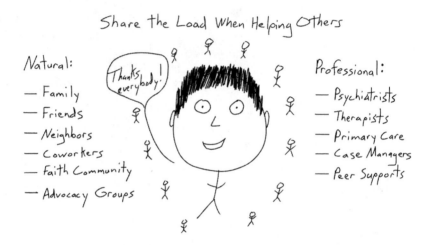

A Note about Confidentiality

As a family member or friend, you are not bound by state or federal rules surrounding patient confidentiality. For example, HIPAA privacy rules do not affect your ability to share important information with professionals in the situation of addressing medication nonadherence or a safety concern. You can always leave a detailed message for a therapist or doctor if you have something meaningful to share about a loved one.

A Story about a Depressed Friend

Suzie was thirty-five years old and had gone through a recent divorce. Her kids alternated weeks with her and her ex-husband. This was her week without the kids, which was five percent relief and ninety-five percent misery. When she didn't have the kids, she didn't get out of bed except to go to work and didn't eat much or exercise. Suzie had experienced her first episode of depression in tenth grade. The depression went away by the end of her junior year of high school and didn't hit her again until shortly after the birth of her twin boys. An antidepressant relieved her postpartum depression and kept her out of depression until this past year, when it no longer seemed to help. Her best friend Ann knew all this. Ann was Suzie's biggest support and Suzie didn't feel she would have survived without her friend's availability, support, and encouragement.

Suzie felt like she had become Ann's "project," which she hated and appreciated at the same time. Over the past month, Ann had started calling her every day when Suzie's kids were with their dad. Ann would not give up. The phone call usually came by 9 a.m. and the questions were often the same. It usually went something like this: "Hi Suzie, are you up? Be honest, are you in bed or out of bed? Get out of bed! I'm swinging by your apartment at ten so we can go for our walk. Hurry up! You have a lot to do before I get there. I'm not getting off the phone until you are out of bed. Okay? Thanks! See you soon!"

Ann was so convinced that Suzie's depression would get better, it seemed like she had been brainwashed by a cult. Ann had even roped other friends and Suzie's sister into connecting with Suzie on her days off. Ann was persistent in asking what Suzie's doctor was doing with her meds, if she was taking her medication and if she was being honest with her doctor and therapist about how she was doing. She even called Suzie's therapist and ratted Suzie out when she tried to hide in bed all day last Saturday. Ann was constantly sharing stories about new treatments for depression and articles that she thought would be encouraging. The thing that felt a bit unbelievable to Suzie was that it seemed like the things Ann was getting her to do were actually starting to work.

You Can Help Friends and Family Who Suffer from Depression

There is no need to feel helpless in the face of others' depression. Despite resistance, you can help your loved ones. Meeting them where they are and nudging them to start taking healthy steps is a reasonable starting place. They may have forgotten all the things that can help them, and you can be the person to remind them that there is always a legitimate reason for hope, holding on, and persevering—no matter how dark the depression is. You can hold on to hope for them and remind them of things that work. Your persistent encouragement and regularly checking in with them will make a difference. Your active involvement and connection to them are meaningful, and your efforts to connect them to others who are willing to help will encourage them until they can do it for themselves.

Reflection

- Read Galatians 6:2. What do you think it means to carry each other's burdens? Do you think this applies to depression?

- What thoughts do you have about IS PATH WARM?

- Was there anything in this chapter that added to your understanding of how to help someone who is depressed? If so, what?

- Are there any steps that you plan to take as a result of reading this chapter (for example, connecting with a friend or family member you have been concerned about, asking a depressed loved one point-blank if they have been experiencing thoughts of suicide, or reviewing the chapter on safety planning)?

Conclusion

Climbing Out Of Depression and Nurturing Your Spiritual Life

But he said to me, "My grace is sufficient for you, for my power is made perfect in weakness." Therefore I will boast all the more gladly about my weaknesses, so that Christ's power may rest on me. That is why, for Christ's sake, I delight in weaknesses, in insults, in hardships, in persecutions, in difficulties. For when I am weak, then I am strong. (2 Corinthians 12:9–10)

Hanging on to Your Spiritual Life

IT IS COMMON TO feel very isolated from God in the midst of your depression. While this is not true for everyone, depression often crowds out all other areas of your life, including your spiritual life. In chapter 11, I shared the concept of your life being like a painter's canvas that the depression is constantly trying to fill. It takes active effort to fill your life canvas with activities and relationships that are meaningful and that will essentially push out the depression.

In depression, it is especially important to pay attention to your relationship with God. As depression often causes low motivation and energy, it can lead people to be less engaged in their spiritual lives. Many people who are severely depressed are either not connected or else they feel isolated despite being connected with others and their church. Even amidst depression, it is essential that you nurture your relationship with God and other Christians.

For some Christians, this is very hard to do while they are depressed. If this sounds like you, then you will need to return to uplifting spiritual activities such as going to church services, reading the Bible, and praying. You can receive encouragement and also encourage others through any number of activities, including:

- Being an active part of your church community by attending worship services.

- Joining a Bible study or prayer group.

- Setting aside time to read the Bible and pray.

- Meeting with your pastor, spiritual director, Christian mentor, or accountability partner.

Pray and Then Access the Care That God Has Made Available

I started this book by talking about the importance of prayer, and I believe it is appropriate to finish with prayer. There is medical research on the positive effects of prayer. The research available suggests that person-to-person prayer has a significant effect on depression[1] and that benefit is maintained a full year later.[2] The available data regarding the effects of prayer on depression are promising. If you have depression, I want to encourage you to pray (and have others pray for you and with you) and then take action by accessing the care God has made available to you.

Depression Is Treatable

Depression is common, and it hits Christians and non-Christians alike. An aspect that can make depression harder on Christians is stigma, which causes unnecessary shame and blocks and delays Christians from accessing effective treatments for depression. It is important to be on the alert as there are many unhelpful and incorrect myths about depression. Depression can be reliably diagnosed, and emotional pain is real. Spiritual battles can occur

---

1. Boelens et al., "Randomized Trial," 382–89.
2. Boelens et al., "Effect of Prayer on Depression and Anxiety," 90–96.

in depression; therefore, getting rid of depression will help you to have the motivation and energy to confront the enemy.

Depression is not your fault, but it is your responsibility to do something effective about it.

In this book, I have covered many strategies and tools for dealing with depression. There is even more information available at my website (lenlantz.com/unJoy). Effective treatments and strategies are provided by God for you. In the same way he has provided insulin to treat diabetes and inhalers to treat asthma, God has provided many natural and medical interventions for depression. Perhaps more importantly, God has provided people—skilled professionals who will genuinely care about you and what you are going through—to help you be equipped to get out of the depression and stay out.

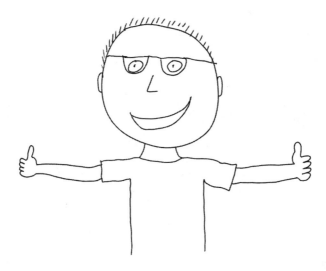

I'm congratulating you for reading through this book and applying what you learned.

You can get through this. Depression can improve greatly, and life will look much better when this happens. I want to encourage you to not give up. Don't be afraid to try something new or work with someone new if you are not seeing improvement or not experiencing the hope and joy that you know you had in the past.

Do you remember Jeff, the strong Christian from chapter 1? He had struggled with severe depression for seventy years. When he finally got the correct treatment and reached remission, he said, "You have *no idea* what it feels like to *not* be depressed!" If he could get better, so can you.

At the start of this book, I stated that this is not a self-help book. It is a get-help book. I have personally witnessed people who have had decades of depression and an extensive trauma history get fully free from depression and stay free. If it was possible for them, it is possible for you, too.

Reflection

- Read 2 Corinthians 12:9–10. Do you think the "weakness" also applies to depression? Do you find this verse encouraging? Why?

- What are the top three things you learned from this book?

- Do you have more hope for yourself or others? Do you feel better equipped to deal with depression for yourself or others?

- Do you feel less of a need to hide your depression?

- What steps did you take as you read this book?

- I said that this is not a self-help book and instead it is a get-help book. Do you agree? Why or why not?

- Do you have a plan to get help for yourself or help others?

- Can you think of any barriers that you will need to overcome that could prevent you from using the ideas from this book to help yourself or others?

- What is one step that you could complete before going to bed tonight?

Resources

Do you remember in chapter 5 when I said, "Don't go it alone?" I mean that. The following resources are for you to use with your team of professionals, *not for you to diagnose yourself or try to treat mental health conditions on your own.*

One of the first things I want to remind you to do is to go to my website (lenlantz.com/unJoy) to access some of the resources and articles mentioned in the text.

Here I have included the following tools:

- Patient Health Questionnaire-9 (PHQ-9).

- Mood Disorder Questionnaire (MDQ).

- Generalized Anxiety Disorder-7 (GAD-7).

- Safety Plan from the Safety Planning Intervention (SPI).

PATIENT HEALTH QUESTIONNAIRE-9 (PHQ-9)

Over the <u>last 2 weeks</u>, how often have you been bothered by any of the following problems? *(Use "✔" to indicate your answer)*	Not at all	Several days	More than half the days	Nearly every day
1. Little interest or pleasure in doing things	0	1	2	3
2. Feeling down, depressed, or hopeless	0	1	2	3
3. Trouble falling or staying asleep, or sleeping too much	0	1	2	3
4. Feeling tired or having little energy	0	1	2	3
5. Poor appetite or overeating	0	1	2	3
6. Feeling bad about yourself — or that you are a failure or have let yourself or your family down	0	1	2	3
7. Trouble concentrating on things, such as reading the newspaper or watching television	0	1	2	3
8. Moving or speaking so slowly that other people could have noticed? Or the opposite — being so fidgety or restless that you have been moving around a lot more than usual	0	1	2	3
9. Thoughts that you would be better off dead or of hurting yourself in some way	0	1	2	3

FOR OFFICE CODING ___0___ + _____ + _____ + _____

=Total Score: _____

If you checked off <u>any</u> problems, how <u>difficult</u> have these problems made it for you to do your work, take care of things at home, or get along with other people?

Not difficult at all	Somewhat difficult	Very difficult	Extremely difficult
☐	☐	☐	☐

Developed by Drs. Robert L. Spitzer, Janet B. W. Williams, Kurt Kroenke, and colleagues, with an educational grant from Pfizer Inc. No permission is required to reproduce, translate, display, or distribute.

Patient Health Questionnaire-9 (PHQ-9): This tool can reveal the severity of depressive symptoms. It can also help you to keep track of your progress in your treatment. You should always review your completed scale with your primary care physician or mental health professional. Here are what the total scores might mean:

- Minimal or no depression (0–4).
- Mild depression (5–9).
- Moderate depression (10–14).
- Moderately severe depression (15–19).
- Severe depression (20–27).

The Mood Disorder Questionnaire (MDQ)

1. Has there ever been a period of time when you were not your usual self and...

   ...you felt so good or so hyper that other people thought you were not your
   normal self or you were so hyper that you got into trouble? ☐ Yes *or* ☐ No

   ...you were so irritable that you shouted at people or started fights or
   arguments? ☐ Yes *or* ☐ No

   ...you felt much more self-confident than usual? ☐ Yes *or* ☐ No

   ...you got much less sleep than usual and found you didn't really miss it? ☐ Yes *or* ☐ No

   ...you were much more talkative or spoke much faster than usual? ☐ Yes *or* ☐ No

   ...thoughts raced through your head or you couldn't slow your mind
   down? ☐ Yes *or* ☐ No

   ...you were so easily distracted by things around you that you had trouble
   concentrating or staying on track? ☐ Yes *or* ☐ No

   ...you had much more energy than usual? ☐ Yes *or* ☐ No

   ...you were much more active or did many more things than usual? ☐ Yes *or* ☐ No

   ...you were much more social or outgoing than usual, for example, you
   telephoned friends in the middle of the night? ☐ Yes *or* ☐ No

   ...you were much more interested in sex than usual? ☐ Yes *or* ☐ No

   ...you did things that were unusual for you or that other people might have
   thought were excessive, foolish, or risky? ☐ Yes *or* ☐ No

   ...spending money got you or your family into trouble? ☐ Yes *or* ☐ No

2. If you checked YES to more than 1 of the above, have several of these ever happened
   during the same period of time? ☐ Yes *or* ☐ No

3. How much of a problem did any of these cause you—like being unable to work; having family,
   money, or legal troubles; getting into arguments or fights? *Please check one response only.*
   ☐ No problem   ☐ Minor problem   ☐ Moderate problem   ☐ Serious problem

Used with permission, granted by Dr. Robert M. A. Hirschfeld.

The Mood Disorder Questionnaire (MDQ): This tool is used to screen for
bipolar disorder. You should always review your completed scale with your
primary care physician or mental health professional. It is strongly recommended that you obtain additional professional assessment for bipolar
disorder if you:

- Answer Yes to seven or more of the events in question #1, *and*

- Answer Yes to question #2, *and*

- Select "Moderate problem" or "Serious problem" for question #3.

GAD-7

Over the <u>last 2 weeks</u>, how often have you been bothered by the following problems? *(Use "✔" to indicate your answer)*	Not at all	Several days	More than half the days	Nearly every day
1. Feeling nervous, anxious or on edge	0	1	2	3
2. Not being able to stop or control worrying	0	1	2	3
3. Worrying too much about different things	0	1	2	3
4. Trouble relaxing	0	1	2	3
5. Being so restless that it is hard to sit still	0	1	2	3
6. Becoming easily annoyed or irritable	0	1	2	3
7. Feeling afraid as if something awful might happen	0	1	2	3

(For office coding: Total Score T____ = ____ + ____ + ____)

Developed by Drs. Robert L. Spitzer, Janet B. W. Williams, Kurt Kroenke, and colleagues, with an educational grant from Pfizer Inc. No permission is required to reproduce, translate, display or distribute.

Generalized Anxiety Disorder-7 (GAD-7): This tool is a standard way of measuring your level of overall anxiety. You should always review your completed scale with your primary care physician or mental health professional. Here are what the total scores might mean:

- Minimal or no anxiety (0–4).
- Mild anxiety (5–9).
- Moderate anxiety (10–14).
- Severe anxiety (15–21).

STANLEY - BROWN SAFETY PLAN

STEP 1: WARNING SIGNS:

1. ....
2. ....
3. ....

STEP 2: INTERNAL COPING STRATEGIES – THINGS I CAN DO TO TAKE MY MIND OFF MY PROBLEMS WITHOUT CONTACTING ANOTHER PERSON:

1. ....
2. ....
3. ....

STEP 3: PEOPLE AND SOCIAL SETTINGS THAT PROVIDE DISTRACTION:

1. Name: _____   Contact: _____

2. Name: _____   Contact: _____

3. Place: _____   4. Place: _____

STEP 4: PEOPLE WHOM I CAN ASK FOR HELP DURING A CRISIS:

1. Name: _____   Contact: _____

2. Name: _____   Contact: _____

3. Name: _____   Contact: _____

STEP 5: PROFESSIONALS OR AGENCIES I CAN CONTACT DURING A CRISIS:

1. Clinician/Agency Name: _____   Phone: _____
Emergency Contact : _____

2. Clinician/Agency Name: _____   Phone: _____
Emergency Contact : _____

3. Local Emergency Department: _____
Emergency Department Address: _____
Emergency Department Phone : _____

4. Suicide Prevention Lifeline Phone: 1-800-273-TALK (8255)

STEP 6: MAKING THE ENVIRONMENT SAFER (PLAN FOR LETHAL MEANS SAFETY):

1. ....
2. ....

Stanley-Brown
Safety Planning Intervention

Used with permission, granted by Drs. Barbara Stanley and Gregory K. Brown.

Safety Plan from the Safety Planning Intervention (SPI): This tool can save your life. Please fill it out completely, make it as detailed as possible, and remember where you put it. Pull out this plan and start following the steps if you are feeling suicidal or if you experience a common trigger for suicidal thoughts. This plan is meant to be updated and improved as you figure out what strategies work the best in helping you to remain safe.

Bibliography

aan het Rot, Marije, et al. "Safety and Efficacy of Repeated-Dose Intravenous Ketamine for Treatment-Resistant Depression." *Biological Psychiatry* 67.2 (2010) 139–45.

Akhtar, Sadaf, and Jane Barlow. "Forgiveness Therapy for the Promotion of Mental Well-Being: A Systematic Review and Meta-Analysis." *Trauma, Violence & Abuse* 19.1 (2018) 107–22.

Babyak, Michael, et al. "Exercise Treatment for Major Depression: Maintenance of Therapeutic Benefit at 10 Months." *Psychosomatic Medicine* 62.5 (2000) 633–38.

Blumenthal, James A., et al. "Effects of Exercise Training on Older Patients with Major Depression." *Archives of Internal Medicine* 159.19 (1999) 2349–56.

———. "Exercise and Pharmacotherapy in the Treatment of Major Depressive Disorder." *Psychosomatic Medicine* 69.7 (2007) 587–96.

Boden, Joseph M., and David M. Fergusson. "Alcohol and Depression." *Addiction* 106.5 (2011) 906–14.

Boden, Joseph M., et al. "Cigarette Smoking and Depression: Tests of Causal Linkages Using a Longitudinal Birth Cohort." *British Journal of Psychiatry* 196.6 (2010) 440–46.

Boelens, Peter A., et al. "The Effect of Prayer on Depression and Anxiety: Maintenance of Positive Influence One Year after Prayer Intervention." *International Journal of Psychiatry in Medicine* 43.1 (2012) 85–98.

———. "A Randomized Trial of the Effect of Prayer on Depression and Anxiety." *International Journal of Psychiatry in Medicine* 39.4 (2009) 377–92.

Brinsley, Jacinta, et al. "Effects of Yoga on Depressive Symptoms in People with Mental Disorders: A Systematic Review and Meta-Analysis." *British Journal of Sports Medicine* 55.17 (2021) 992–1000.

Burns, David D. *Feeling Good.* 2nd ed. New York: Harper, 2000.

Cole, Eleanor J., et al. "Stanford Accelerated Intelligent Neuromodulation Therapy for Treatment-Resistant Depression." *American Journal of Psychiatry* 177.8 (2020) 716–26.

———. "Stanford Neuromodulation Therapy (SNT): A Double-Blind Randomized Controlled Trial." *American Journal of Psychiatry* 179.2 (2022) 132–41.

Bibliography

Cuijpers, Pim, et al. "The Efficacy of Non-Directive Supportive Therapy for Adult Depression: A Meta-Analysis." *Clinical Psychology Review* 32.4 (2012) 280–91.

Daly, Ella J., et al. "Efficacy and Safety of Intranasal Esketamine Adjunctive to Oral Antidepressant Therapy in Treatment-Resistant Depression: A Randomized Clinical Trial." *JAMA Psychiatry* 75.2 (2018) 139–48.

Davis, Alan K., et al. "Effects of Psilocybin-Assisted Therapy on Major Depressive Disorder: A Randomized Clinical Trial." *JAMA Psychiatry* 78.5 (2021) 481–89.

Dunner, David L., et al. "A Multisite, Naturalistic, Observational Study of Transcranial Magnetic Stimulation for Patients with Pharmacoresistant Major Depressive Disorder: Durability of Benefit over a 1-Year Follow-Up Period." *Journal of Clinical Psychiatry* 75.12 (2014) 1394–1401.

Florentine, Julia B., and Catherine Crane. "Suicide Prevention by Limiting Access to Methods: A Review of Theory and Practice." *Social Science & Medicine* 70.10 (2010) 1626–32.

Gortner, Eric T., et al. "Cognitive-Behavioral Treatment for Depression: Relapse Prevention." *Journal of Consulting and Clinical Psychology* 66.2 (1998) 377–84.

Gregory, Robert J., et al. "Cognitive Bibliotherapy for Depression: A Meta-Analysis." *Professional Psychology: Research and Practice* 35.3 (2004) 275–80.

Hankerson, Sidney H., et al. "Ministers' Perceptions of Church-Based Programs to Provide Depression Care for African Americans." *Journal of Urban Health* 90.4 (2013) 685–98.

Heinemann, Linda V., and Torsten Heinemann. "Burnout Research: Emergence and Scientific Investigation of a Contested Diagnosis." *SAGE Open* (January 2017) 1–12. https://doi.org/10.1177/2158244017697154.

Hengartner, Michael P., et al. "Efficacy of New-Generation Antidepressants Assessed with the Montgomery-Asberg Depression Rating Scale, the Gold Standard Clinician Rating Scale: A Meta-Analysis of Randomised Placebo-Controlled Trials." *PLOS One* 15.2 (February 2020) 1–11. https://doi.org/10.1371/journal.pone.0229381.

Hoffman, Benson M., et al. "Exercise and Pharmacotherapy in Patients with Major Depression: One-Year Follow-Up of the SMILE Study." *Psychosomatic Medicine* 73.2 (2011) 127–33.

Horvath, Adam O., and B. Dianne Symonds. "Relation Between Working Alliance and Outcome in Psychotherapy: A Meta-Analysis." *Journal of Counseling Psychology* 38.2 (1991) 139–49.

Isserles, Moshe, et al. "Cognitive–Emotional Reactivation During Deep Transcranial Magnetic Stimulation over the Prefrontal Cortex of Depressive Patients Affects Antidepressant Outcome." *Journal of Affective Disorders* 128.3 (2011) 235–42.

James-Palmer, Aurora, et al. "Yoga as an Intervention for the Reduction of Symptoms of Anxiety and Depression in Children and Adolescents: A Systematic Review." *Frontiers in Pediatrics* 8.78 (March 2020) 1–16. https://doi.org/10.3389/fped.2020.00078.

Janssen, Clemens W., et al. "Whole-Body Hyperthermia for the Treatment of Major Depressive Disorder: A Randomized Clinical Trial." *JAMA Psychiatry* 73.8 (2016) 789–95.

Karyotaki, Eirini, et al. "Efficacy of Self-Guided Internet-Based Cognitive Behavioral Therapy in the Treatment of Depressive Symptoms: A Meta-Analysis of Individual Participant Data." *JAMA Psychiatry* 74.4 (2017) 351–59.

Bibliography

Kelly, Michael S., et al. "Initial Response to Transcranial Magnetic Stimulation Treatment for Depression Predicts Subsequent Response." *Journal of Neuropsychiatry and Clinical Neurosciences* 29.2 (2017) 179–82.

Kendall, R. T. *Total Forgiveness*. Lake Mary, FL: Charisma House, 2007.

Kessler, Ronald C., et al. "Lifetime Prevalence and Age-of-Onset Distributions of DSM-IV Disorders in the National Comorbidity Survey Replication." *Archives of General Psychiatry* 62.6 (2005) 593–602.

Koenig, Harold G., et al. "Religiously-Integrated Cognitive Behavioural Therapy for Major Depression in Chronic Medical Illness: Review of Results from a Randomized Clinical Trial." *Health and Social Care Chaplaincy* 4.2 (2016) 237–53. https://doi.org/10.1558/hscc.v4i2.31655.

Kraus, Christoph, et al. "Prognosis and Improved Outcomes in Major Depression: A Review." *Translational Psychiatry* 9.127 (2019) 1–17. https://doi.org/10.1038/s41398-019-0460-3.

Krupnick, Janice L., et al. "The Role of the Therapeutic Alliance in Psychotherapy and Pharmacotherapy Outcome: Findings in the National Institute of Mental Health Treatment of Depression Collaborative Research Program." *Journal of Consulting and Clinical Psychology* 64.3 (1996) 532–39.

Lam, Raymond W., et al. "The Can-SAD Study: A Randomized Controlled Trial of the Effectiveness of Light Therapy and Fluoxetine in Patients with Winter Seasonal Affective Disorder." *American Journal of Psychiatry* 163.5 (2006) 805–12.

Lambert, Michael J., et al. "The Effects of Providing Therapists with Feedback on Patient Progress During Psychotherapy: Are Outcomes Enhanced?" *Psychotherapy Research* 11.1 (2001) 49–68.

Lantz, Len. "Light Therapy for Depression: Are You Doing It Right?" https://psychiatryresource.com/articles/light-therapy.

———. "Stigma and 7 Million American Christians with Depression." https://psychiatryresource.com/articles/stigma-and-7-million-depressed-christians.

Lewis, C. S. *Collected Letters: Vol. 3*. Edited by Walter Hooper. London: HarperCollins, 2007.

Mazzucchelli, Trevor, et al. "Behavioral Activation Treatments for Depression in Adults: A Meta-Analysis and Review." *Clinical Psychology: Science and Practice* 16.4 (2009) 383–411.

Miller, Scott D., et al. "The Outcome of Psychotherapy: Yesterday, Today, and Tomorrow." *Psychotherapy* 50.1 (2013) 88–97.

Möller, Hans-Jürgen. "Outcomes in Major Depressive Disorder: The Evolving Concept of Remission and Its Implications for Treatment." *The World Journal of Biological Psychiatry* 9.2 (2008) 102–14.

National Center for Health Statistics. "International Classification of Diseases, Tenth Revision, Clinical Modification (ICD-10-CM)." https://ftp.cdc.gov/pub/Health_Statistics/NCHS/Publications/ICD10CM/2022/icd10cm_codes_2022.txt.

Obisesan, Olufunmilayo H., et al. "Association Between e-Cigarette Use and Depression in the Behavioral Risk Factor Surveillance System, 2016–2017." *JAMA Network Open* 2.12 (2019) 1–11. https://doi.org/10.1001/jamanetworkopen.2019.16800.

Onaemo, Vivian N., et al. "Comorbid Cannabis Use Disorder with Major Depression and Generalized Anxiety Disorder: A Systematic Review with Meta-Analysis of Nationally Representative Epidemiological Surveys." *Journal of Affective Disorders* 281 (2021) 467–75.

Bibliography

Packer, J. I. *Knowing God*. Downers Grove: InterVarsity, 1973.

Peteet, John R. "Approaching Religiously Reinforced Mental Health Stigma: A Conceptual Framework." *Psychiatric Services* 70.9 (2019) 846–48.

Pingleton, Jared, et al. "Study of Acute Mental Illness and Christian Faith." https://lifewayresearch.com/wp-content/uploads/2014/09/Acute-Mental-Illness-and-Christian-Faith-Research-Report-1.pdf.

Pitman, Alexandra L., et al. "Bereavement by Suicide as a Risk Factor for Suicide Attempt: A Cross-Sectional National UK-Wide Study of 3432 Young Bereaved Adults." *BMJ Open* 6.1 (2016) 1–11. http://dx.doi.org/10.1136/bmjopen-2015-009948.

Pizzagalli, Diego A. "Frontocingulate Dysfunction in Depression: Toward Biomarkers of Treatment Response." *Neuropsychopharmacology* 36.1 (2011) 183–206.

Prudic, Joan, et al. "Effectiveness of Electroconvulsive Therapy in Community Settings." *Biological Psychiatry* 55.3 (2004) 301–12.

Ramel, Wiveka, et al. "The Effects of Mindfulness Meditation on Cognitive Processes and Affect in Patients with Past Depression." *Cognitive Therapy and Research* 28.4 (2004) 433–55.

Reese, Robert J., et al. "Does a Continuous Feedback System Improve Psychotherapy Outcome?" *Psychotherapy: Theory, Research, Practice, Training* 46.4 (2009) 418–31.

Ruhrmann, S., et al. "Effects of Fluoxetine versus Bright Light in the Treatment of Seasonal Affective Disorder." *Psychological Medicine* 28.4 (1998) 923–33.

Smith, Nancy M., et al. "Three-Year Follow-Up of Bibliotherapy for Depression." *Journal of Consulting and Clinical Psychology* 65.2 (1997) 324–27.

Stanley, Barbara, and Gregory K. Brown. "Safety Planning Intervention: A Brief Intervention to Mitigate Suicide Risk." *Cognitive and Behavioral Practice* 19.2 (2012) 256–64.

Takahashi, Yoshitomo. "Depression and Suicide." *Journal of the Japan Medical Association* 44.8 (2001) 359–63.

Wall, Christopher A., et al. "Neurocognitive Effects of Repetitive Transcranial Magnetic Stimulation in Adolescents with Major Depressive Disorder." *Frontiers in Psychiatry* 4.165 (December 2013) 1–8. https://doi.org/10.3389/fpsyt.2013.00165.

Watkins, Edward R., et al. "Rumination-Focused Cognitive–Behavioural Therapy for Residual Depression: Phase II Randomised Controlled Trial." *The British Journal of Psychiatry* 199.4 (2011) 317–22.

Watt, Jeffrey R. "Calvin on Suicide." *Church History* 66.3 (1997) 463–76. https://doi.org/10.2307/3169451.

Wesselmann, Eric D., et al. "Religious Beliefs about Mental Illness Influence Social Support Preferences." *Journal of Prevention & Intervention in the Community* 43.3 (2015) 165–74.

Wilcox, Holly C., et al. "Psychiatric Morbidity, Violent Crime, and Suicide Among Children and Adolescents Exposed to Parental Death." *Journal of the American Academy of Child & Adolescent Psychiatry* 49.5 (2010) 514–23.

Williams, Leanne M. "Precision Psychiatry: A Neural Circuit Taxonomy for Depression and Anxiety." *Lancet Psychiatry* 3.5 (2016) 472–80.

Made in the USA
Las Vegas, NV
31 March 2024